CBD

HANDBOOK

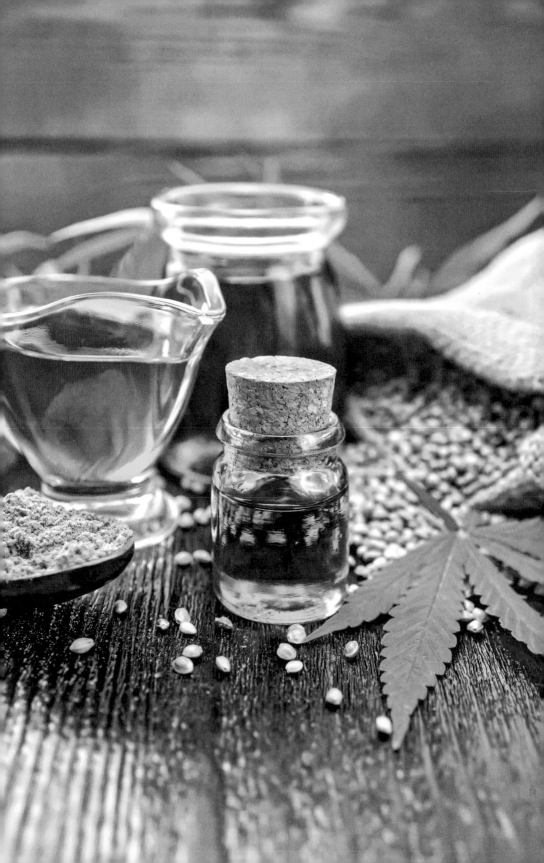

Recipes for Natural Living

CBD

HANDBOOK

BARBARA BROWNELL GROGAN

Foreword by **Deanna Gabriel Vierck, CCH, CN**

STERLING
New York

STERLING
New York

An Imprint of Sterling Publishing Co., Inc.
1166 Avenue of the Americas
New York, NY 10036

ISBN 978-1-4549-3465-3

Distributed in Canada by Sterling Publishing Co., Inc.
c/o Canadian Manda Group, 664 Annette Street
Toronto, Ontario M6S 2C8, Canada
Distributed in the United Kingdom by GMC Distribution Services
Castle Place, 166 High Street, Lewes, East Sussex BN7 1XU, England
Distributed in Australia by NewSouth Books
University of New South Wales, Sydney, NSW 2052, Australia

For information about custom editions, special sales,
and premium and corporate purchases, please
contact Sterling Special Sales at 800-805-5489
or specialsales@sterlingpublishing.com.

Manufactured in Canada

2 4 6 8 10 9 7 5 3 1

sterlingpublishing.com

Cover design by Elizabeth Mihaltse Lindy
Interior design by Christine Heun

For image credits—see page 229

CONTENTS

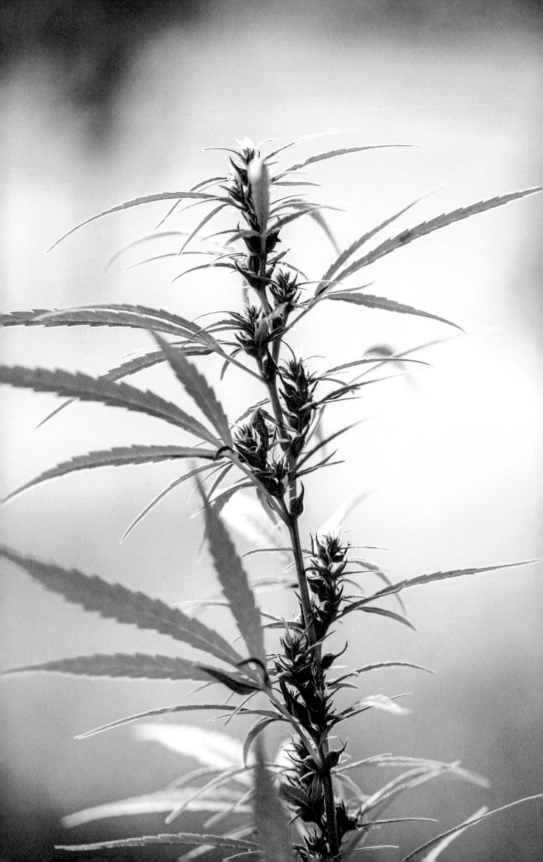

FOREWORD

As an herbalist of nearly 15 years and a lifelong lover of plants, I have many plants that are near and dear to my heart. I'm constantly amazed by the incredible healing benefits found in powerful plant allies, and one plant that holds a special place in my heart is hemp. I feel such deep gratitude for this plant. It was nearly two years ago that I began consistent use of a non-psychoactive CBD supplement made from hemp rather than marijuana. My results were so fantastic that my husband also began regular supplementation, and I can honestly say that this plant has changed our lives. I was in a state of chronic stress, fatigue, and irritation, and it was affecting my relationships. My inner world was getting toxic. My husband was continually injuring his back, leaving him immobile for more than a week at a time. We were a mess! When I think back to those days and compare them to our current reality, the difference is shocking. I no longer experience regular stress-related outbursts. My inner voice has gotten much kinder, and my husband hasn't thrown his back out in nearly two years. While this transformation was occurring for my family, I was witnessing hundreds of people supplementing with CBD for a wide variety of acute and chronic ailments—physical, mental, emotional. Most of these individuals enjoyed fantastic relief as a result of the incredible healing properties of the hemp plant.

There are many historical references about the use of marijuana as medicine but fewer references to the variety of cannabis discussed in this book: hemp. Why has there been such an eruption of excitement over the medicinal benefits of hemp in modern days? Hemp naturally contains larger amounts of cannabidiol (CBD), which offers healing without marijuana's THC-induced "high."

I believe this benevolent plant is providing relief for a crisis created by modern lifestyles—one that has caused levels of emotional and physical stress to reach an all-time high. The constant exposure to environmental toxins from vehicles, industrial farming, and herbicides/pesticides for lawncare is off the charts. The impacts from the decline in the general standard of nutrition over the last few decades, combined with constant stimulation from electronics and expectations that we be master multitaskers, are increasingly problematic. Chronic ailments are widespread, along with depression, anxiety, and a general attitude of being overwhelmed. We are often described as a society of overstimulated, undernourished, lonely people who are expected to perform at high levels. What does all this have to do with hemp? All of these experiences negatively impact the function of our endocannabinoid system (ECS). When this important system can't do its job properly, the list of emotional, mental, and physical ailments that result is very long.

In this book you will learn how the endocannabinoid system plays a large role in the proper function of important body systems such as the endocrine, immune, reproductive, and digestive. It assists in the smooth operation of detoxification pathways and has huge impacts on our mental/emotional health. In fact, as scientists study this system more deeply, they're learning that the ECS is a master regulatory system in the human body, and when it can't work properly, we suffer some very uncomfortable consequences. Why is this system experiencing such challenges in the modern day? The ECS is stimulated by a state of relaxed nourishment. It, like all systems in the human body, operates on well-digested nutrients and flows when an individual is calm and relaxed. The ECS thrives in states of gratitude, love, inspiration, and community connection. The realities of the modern lifestyle have caused a severe drop in the ECS function for many because the aforementioned elements are often absent. This makes the need to supplement greater than ever before. This need for supplementation makes the hemp plant, rich in compounds that nourish the ECS, an incredibly valuable plant ally.

Estimations about the future value of the hemp industry, often reported to be multiple billions of dollars by 2025, reflect a population of people hungry for access to this plant. Over the last ten or more years, there has been a growing acceptance of marijuana as medicine. Many have provided testimonials about miraculous healing experienced as a result of the plant's therapeutic properties, which sparked a wave of research and clinical trials to discover more about the healing compounds in marijuana. Through this, we learned about CBD's power. This plant compound showed great potential, and people began to look to hemp rather than marijuana due to its larger amount of non-psychoactive CBD and the absence of legal restrictions that surround its sister plant. Fast-forward a few years to the current CBD craze. Everyone seems interested in exploring the benefits of CBD supplements, and this growing curiosity and demand have stimulated the emergence of one of the biggest, most exciting industries of our lifetime. This is just the beginning.

In this book, Barbara Brownell Grogan offers clarity on a subject that can often seem confusing. She's taken information from the industry's leading experts and distilled it into an offering that will satisfy both the novice and the experienced hemp connoisseur. Barbara walks her readers through the confusing process of selecting the right CBD product by explaining the various forms of hemp supplements and the benefits attributed to each. And to make the whole experience more creative and fun, she has offered a collection of recipes that are delicious, nourishing, and full of powerfully beneficial ingredients to complement hemp's incredible healing abilities. It has been an honor and a pleasure to take this journey with Barbara, and I am confident that you will feel the same as you explore the information offered in these pages. I'm extremely excited about the positive impact this plant medicine can have on our world, and I'm deeply grateful to Barbara Brownell Grogan for her beautiful contribution here. After you read this book, I know you'll feel the same.

—**DEANNA GABRIEL VIERCK, CCH, CN,** is a clinical herbalist and transformational healer in Boulder, Colorado. Her private practice focuses on assisting others using energy healing, plant spirit medicines, and flower essences. Visit www.DeannaGabrielVierck.com to learn more.

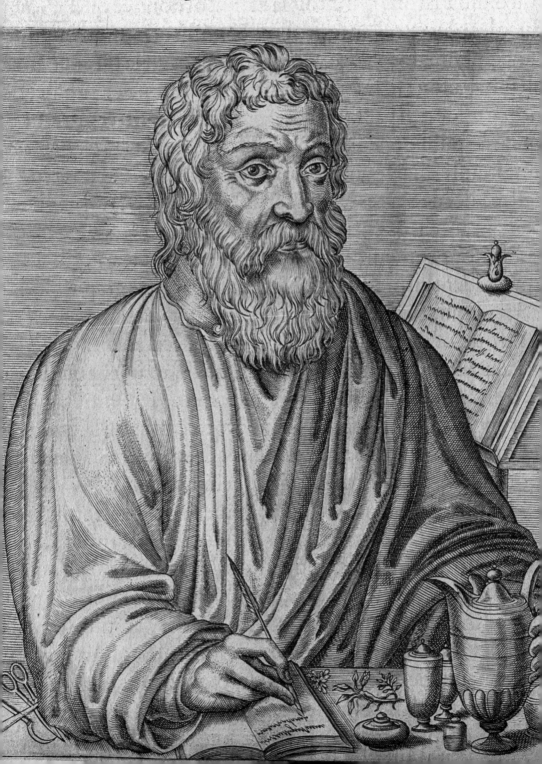

Introduction

In this age of opioid addiction, there is widespread fear of synthetic pharmaceuticals and their toxic, addictive properties. With the ever-increasing understanding of our bodies, our systems, our cells, and our DNA, scientists are working around the clock to develop medicines to support general health and to target vicious invasive diseases and conditions, from arthritis and cancer to hypertension and post-traumatic stress (PTS).

What if scientists could derive an effective medicine from plants rather than synthetics? And what if that medicine were so tried and true that its mother plant had been listed as one of the favorite healers of the Chinese emperor Shen Nung, some 4,700 years ago? Or that its parts were consumed by Siddhartha, the Buddha, in the sixth century BCE and by Hippocrates 100 years later? Or by visionary doctors of the Golden Age of Islam in the ninth century CE and Queen Victoria in the 1800s? What if it were easy to grow, effective, and healing for specific conditions, and it enhanced general well-being?

Many doctors, herbalists, healers, and drug companies believe there is such a medicinal plant. And they believe it has an extraordinary future. It is called hemp. And among its healing plant components is a superstar: cannabidiol, or CBD.

Hemp CBD is a hot topic in healing circles—both mainstream and alternative. You've likely heard about hemp's cousin marijuana becoming legal for medical use because of its healing plant compounds. What makes the two plants different? They come from the same plant family and carry the same healing compound, CBD. But marijuana also has other plant compounds that deliver psychoactive effects; hemp doesn't. For this reason, hemp CBD is gaining warp-speed traction in the medical world. And you need to know about it.

We're writing this book at a milestone in the annals of marijuana-hemp research. You've likely read about—or experienced—marijuana's good effects and bad. You've heard the terms "marijuana" and "hemp" thrown around interchangeably, but you're not really sure what each has to offer. This book will help. It will reveal timely studies, case histories, and federal milestones from the National Institutes of Health, the Mayo Clinic, the Food and Drug Administration, the Department of Health and Human Services, and much more. Its purpose is to set you confidently on your path to using hemp CBD for healing and well-being.

While I am the scribe for this tome, our guiding light is Deanna Gabriel Vierck, CCH, CN, clinical herbalist, nutritionist, and flower essence practitioner. Deanna instructs, lectures, and develops curriculum on holistic living and the part CBD plays in it. Trained as a biologist and botanist, she has a reverence for plants that runs deep. Before CBD blew onto the world stage in a big way, Deanna taught cannabis therapy in the United States and Canada. She also developed salves and massage oils for the medical marijuana business; she went on to create early hemp products for a successful Colorado botanicals business, developing a line that endures today. Now in private practice, Deanna finds CBD "a big plant ally" as she guides clients toward long-term health and well-being. "There's so much interest, curiosity, and hunger to know more about CBD," she says. Throughout the book she'll share insights on CBD that she's gleaned from her personal and professional experience.

HOW TO USE THIS BOOK

Easy and *useful* are the key words for this book. Its intent is to give you succinct information on hemp CBD, to help you identify your potential needs, and to provide recipes for your own journey of learning and healing.

Keep in mind that *The CBD Handbook* is not prescriptive. Always consult your health care provider as you begin your hemp CBD healing journey. Once you've determined together the most beneficial product for your ailment, condition, or search for optimal well-being, you're ready to go. This book is, however, intended to expand your world and introduce you to the herbal healing CBD has to offer. We hope you find its four sections enlightening.

Part One: CBD: The Science and the Story

This section will teach you the basics. It defines and provides the essential background on hemp CBD. First and foremost, it describes the difference between psychoactive marijuana and non-psychoactive hemp. It also explains how hemp CBD oil is different from hemp seed oil—a longstanding ingredient in shampoos and skin lotions. You will also discover the history of the hemp plant and how our body's endocannabinoid system (ECS) works and interacts with CBD.

Part Two: Choosing CBD

Here you will discover the guidelines on choosing the best CBD product for you. You will learn about the different methods used by experts to extract CBD, the most-used supplemental delivery systems, and the potential absorption levels of each kind. You will also learn to read labels and recommended doses, and how to set up your CBD kitchen for healing and wellness.

Part Three: Ailments and Conditions

This section is the nuts and bolts of the book—the go-to reference that should always be within reach. You'll discover five major conditions often considered the source of scores of ailments, acute or chronic. Beyond the five umbrella conditions, you'll discover 35 other conditions for which CBD has been a documented healer. Each part will open with a history of the ailment and the simple science behind it; its triggers; and a range of its time-tested remedies—including CBD. Specific CBD research studies and trials from major clinics, including NIH and Mayo, as well as a few personal—and powerful—testimonials, will back up our words.

Part Four: Healing CBD Recipes

We'll lead you a step beyond buying capsules and gels, into a creative realm with more than 40 recipes that show you how to make the most of hemp CBD to concoct healing drinks, foods, and topicals. The novice CBD user is the focus of the recipes. Each is simple and straightforward, using standard measures and giving you tips for best outcome. All of the recipes promote using natural ingredients that won't counteract CBD's healing effects.

Now, let's begin.

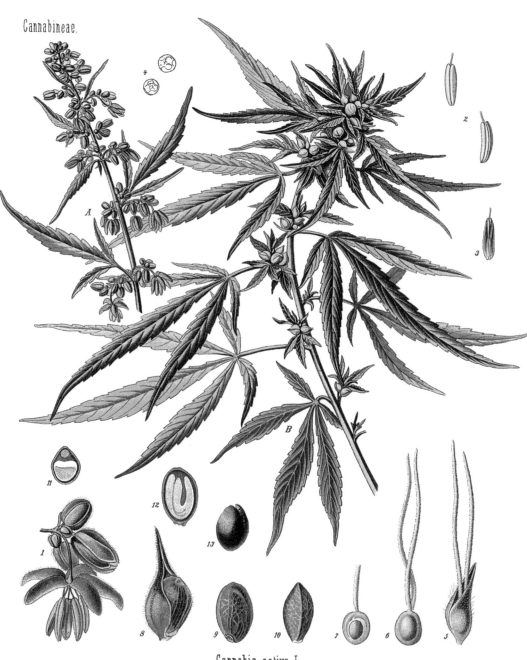

Cannabineae.

Cannabis sativa L.

W. Müller

PART ONE

CBD:
The Science
and the Story

WHAT IS CBD?

Basically, CBD, or cannabidiol (CANN-ah-bid-EYE-awl), is a kind of cannabinoid, or chemical compound. It can be found in both the hemp and the marijuana plants, along with more than 100 other cannabinoids that have healing effects on the body.

Marijuana's CBD is just as healing as hemp's CBD, but here's the hitch: marijuana also carries a high percentage of the intoxicating cannabinoid tetrahydrocannabinol, or THC. Though hemp plants produce THC, the compounds are less prevalent than in marijuana.

When extracting CBD from either plant, there is some THC that comes along—a lot when the CBD is extracted from marijuana, and a little when it comes from hemp. Research has determined that products with more than 0.3 percent THC content can deliver unwanted intoxicating effects. CBD extracted from hemp naturally carries less than 0.3 percent THC—so it is said to deliver healing without the high.

Besides its psychoactive potential, a THC amount greater than 0.3 percent also makes the product illegal in the United States unless you have a license to grow, process, or buy marijuana for medicinal purposes or live in a state where recreational marijuana is legal. On the other hand, hemp CBD can be bought by a wide range of people, without a medical license.

You might say that hemp CBD is all about healing—and that's the focus of this book.

WHAT'S THE DIFFERENCE BETWEEN THE HEMP AND MARIJUANA PLANTS?

Here's a quick botany lesson and a simple diagram: The hemp family of plants (*Cannabaceae*) contains the hemp genus. The hemp genus has one species, called marijuana (*Cannabis sativa*). The marijuana species contains the subspecies *Cannabis sativa*, often called hemp or industrial hemp. There is also a subspecies called *Cannabis indica*, which is often referred to as recreational marijuana or simply marijuana.

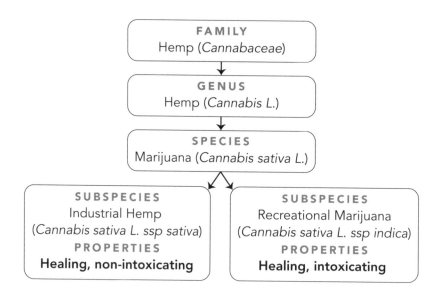

Here's what you need to keep in mind when buying hemp products: while the botanical subspecies above are clearly indicated, product labels may be confusing.

In a marijuana dispensary, for instance, both "sativa" and "indica" may be used for two different categories of THC-potent marijuana. A calming, nighttime product may be labeled "indica," and an energizing, daytime product may be labeled "sativa." Most marijuana bought in a dispensary will claim therapeutic properties from CBD, but be aware: it will likely contain enough THC to cause intoxication.

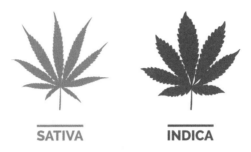

SATIVA   INDICA

On the other hand, when you purchase hemp CBD at a local health food store or online, it was probably extracted from cannabis sativa, but the label will not include this language. Instead it will likely indicate that it is a hemp product that is rich in CBD, with 0.3 percent THC or less. To learn more about labeling, go to page 51.

NOW THAT YOU KNOW ABOUT HEMP, DO YOU BUY HEMP OIL OR HEMP SEED OIL?

You may be thinking: "I've been using hemp seed oil shampoo forever—so what's the big deal?" Here's the difference.

Hemp seed oil, made from the crushed seed of the hemp plant, stocks shelves in many health food stores. It's been a beauty and medicinal staple for centuries—3,000 years in China alone. Healthful omega-3 and omega-6 fatty acids not only boost hair strength and shine but benefit heart disease, high blood pressure, skin disorders, and more. Powerful healing components include gamma-linoleic acids, protein, calcium, iron, and magnesium. But while hemp seed oil gets high marks in the world of natural remedies, it has little to no CBD.

Hemp CBD oil, on the other hand, is produced from the same hemp plant but extracted from the CBD-rich flowers, leaves, and stalks. Besides harboring the same good fats, protein, calcium, and other nutrients found in hemp seed oil, hemp CBD oil has CBD and other cannabinoids, which have the special ability to heal by interacting with the endocannabinoid system within the body. We will dive into this more on pages 16–21.

THE HISTORY OF HEMP

The hemp CBD story begins with the story of hemp—the umbrella for both the hemp and the marijuana plants. For thousands of years, the intoxicating marijuana has been touted as the primary healer. Many scientists and health experts still hold that the healing power of THC combined with CBD is greater than that of CBD alone. Only recently—since the 1940s—has the non-psychoactive hemp plant been held up as its own significant medicine. Let's walk through time and look at both hemp's and marijuana's rich and intertwined histories.

The journey begins as long ago as 40,000 years—perhaps longer—on the Tibetan Plateau. While both subspecies of the hemp plant flourished in the Himalayas, marijuana was likely the go-to healer and spiritual aid. In nearby India it became interwoven with Ayurvedic and Yogic practices. Healers harvested resin or secreted gum from the plant's glands, which covered its leaves and buds, to make the potent product called *hashish*, or hash. From this they made *charas*—a hand-rolled cannabis concentrate enjoyed much like chewing tobacco—to deliver marijuana's healing powers and spiritual highs. From India and environs, the knowledge and use of the hemp plant—both marijuana and hemp—spread east, then west.

In China, hemp's medicinal uses became mainstream during the rule of Emperor Shen Nung, around 2,700 BCE These traditional remedies were passed from generation to generation and finally recorded around the first century CE in perhaps the world's oldest book of plants, or pharmacopeia, the *Pen-ts'ao Ching.*

About 2,500 BCE in ancient Scythia, today parts of eastern Europe, the Greek historian Herodotus recorded observations of marijuana use. He

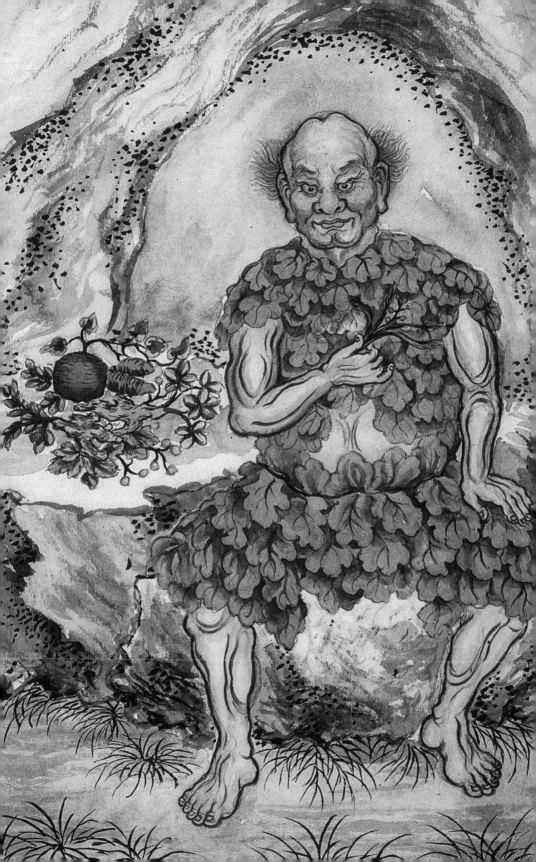

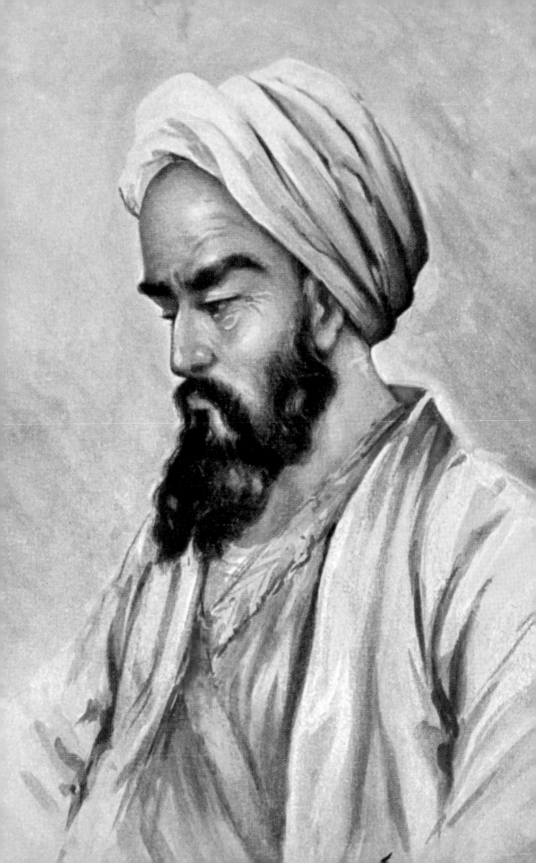

witnessed citizens crawl into a tent where a pile of hot stones glowed at the center. They then "take seed of this [*marijuana*] and . . . throw it on the red-hot stones," he wrote, "where it smoulders and sends forth such fumes that no Greek vapor-bath could surpass it. The Scythians howl in their joy at the vapor-bath." Additionally, extensive research in Romania in the twentieth century uncovered traces of the plant at Bronze Age sites where marijuana may have been used in burial ceremonies.

Back in India, the sacred text *Atharva Veda*, written around 1,400 BCE, describes the soothing effects of the hemp plant, possibly the marijuana variety. And a few centuries later Siddhartha, better known as the Buddha, lived his sacred life on meals consisting primarily of hemp seeds and other plant parts.

Moving westward to Greece at the turn of the millennium, hemp—likely marijuana—caught the eye of revered physician Hippocrates, who praised its healing powers. It later took hold with visionary healers of the Muslim world, such as al-Razi, and likewise became part of their texts.

Around 500 CE, the hemp variety of the plant took a firm roothold in Europe, growing into a staple for Western economy. Healing powers aside, hemp's strong and flexible fibers made it the go-to plant for producing rope and creating canvas for sails to support sea-bound trade and naval ships. (In fact, the term "canvas" comes from "cannabis.") For the same reasons, hemp flourished in the New World later, in the 1600s.

In the 1760s, George Washington touted the hemp plant's resilience and economic importance and grew it at Mount Vernon and his other properties. Hemp was used to make the paper that held early drafts of Thomas Jefferson's Declaration of Independence and the cloth for the first American flags.

But it was Benjamin Franklin who highlighted the non-intoxicating hemp plant as a healer through articles in his *Pennsylvania Gazette*. He touted the seeds as "abating venereal desires" and the leaves as "good against burns."

A medicinal revolution was just around the corner. Beginning in 1839, Irish physician William Brooke O'Shaughnessy spent years in India studying local healing methods. He documented how various parts of the hemp plant—most likely marijuana—addressed maladies from chronic obstructive pulmonary disease (COPD) to neuralgia, guiding doctors to begin with low doses to avoid "hemp inebriation." Upon his return to England, he introduced

A Declaration by the Representatives of the UNITED STATES OF AMERICA, in General Congress assembled.

When in the course of human events it becomes necessary for one people to dissolve the political bands which have connected them with another, and to assume among the powers of the earth the separate and equal station to which the laws of nature & of nature's god entitle them, a decent respect to the opinions of mankind requires that they should declare the causes which impel them to the separation.

We hold these truths to be self-evident; that all men are created equal, that they are endowed by their creator with inherent & inalienable rights; that among these are life, & liberty, & the pursuit of happiness; that to secure these rights, governments are instituted among men, deriving their just powers from the consent of the governed; that whenever any form of government becomes destructive of these ends, it is the right of the people to alter or to abolish it, & to institute new government, laying it's foundation on such principles & organising it's powers in such form, as to them shall seem most likely to effect their safety & happiness. prudence indeed will dictate that governments long established should not be changed for light & transient causes: and accordingly all experience hath shewn that mankind are more disposed to suffer while evils are sufferable, than to right themselves by abolishing the forms to which they are accustomed. but when a long train of abuses & usurpations [begun at a distinguished period, &] pursuing invariably the same object, evinces a design to reduce them under absolute Despotism, it is their right, it is their duty, to throw off such + & to provide new guards for their future security. such has been the patient sufferance of these colonies; & such is now the necessity which constrains them to expunge their former systems of government. the history of the present king of Great Britain. is a history of unremitting injuries and usurpations, [among which, appears no solitary fact to contradict the uniform tenor of the rest [all of which] have] in direct object the establishment of an absolute tyranny over these states. to prove this, let facts be submitted to a candid world, [for the truth of which we pledge a faith yet unsullied by falsehood.]

Dr. Franklin's handwriting

Mr. Adams's handwriting

remedies based on "native" treatments for rheumatism, cholera, tetanus, and seizures, calling it an "anti-convulsive remedy of the greatest value." This value spread quickly to the United States; by 1850, hemp was listed in the *U.S. Pharmacopeia of Medicines and Dietary Supplements*. But this kind of hemp was still the powerful marijuana variety.

One favorite use for this intoxicating hemp was as a candy called Gunjah Wallah Hasheesh, hailed by advertisers as a "nervine," and which held "the true secret of youth and beauty." During the Civil War, General Robert E. Lee found the candy so vital that he wrote: "I wish it was in my power to place a Dollar Box of the HASHEESH CANDY into the pocket of every Confederate Soldier, because I am convinced that it speedily relieves Debility, Fatigue and Suffering." By the turn of the century, the healing power of hemp—the marijuana kind—was being advertised on bottles of *Cannabis Americana* produced by the mega-pharmaceutical company Parke-Davis.

And then the hallowed hemp plant slipped from king to criminal.

In 1906, the United States Congress established the Food and Drug Administration, which demanded clear labeling on all foods and medicines—a great idea. But it triggered a domino effect: it led to ten ingredients, including both marijuana and non-intoxicating hemp varieties, being placed on an "addictive" list. Then, starting in 1910 and continuing through 1920, immigrants escaping the Mexican Revolution brought marijuana into the United States as a recreational product.

Shortly after marijuana's arrival in the States, the Federal Bureau of Narcotics was founded, in 1930. Its officials grouped hemp species under the name "marijuana" and campaigned against their so-called poisonous, debauchery-inducing effects. A witch hunt led by FBN's legendary director Harry Anslinger, aided by newspaper mogul William Randolph Hearst, targeted not only Mexican immigrants, but also African Americans. Even celebrated musician Louis Armstrong was on the hit list. Both plants grew in notoriety, and the differences between them started to blur.

Today both varieties remain on a forbidden list—called Schedule 1 Drugs—established through the Controlled Substance Act of 1970. But changes are happening quickly. The persistence of laboratory scientists, doctors, and other medical experts has led to the legalization of medicinal use for seizures, nausea from chemotherapy, and multiple other ailments. As of June 2018, the FDA has approved an exciting new prescriptive drug containing cannabis, called Epidiolex®, to treat two rare forms of epilepsy.

As of 2018, some 30 states have legalized medical marijuana, meaning products can be purchased if prescribed; and several states, including Alaska, California, and Colorado, as well as Washington, D.C., allow residents over the age of 21 to grow a limited number of marijuana plants for recreational use. Additionally, hemp's growth and use is legal in all 50 states, thanks to the Farm Bill passed in December 2018. While the bill does not fully lift hemp's Schedule 1 status, it does create exceptions that take a major step toward making hemp production mainstream: hemp can be grown as an agricultural plant in all states—with proper licensing; and hemp products can cross state lines—as long as the products are created legally.

So what's next? Through research, ongoing trials, and increased use in the medical world, experts are zeroing in on the science behind the healing components in both varieties. Major medical journals such as the *Journal of the American Medical Association* (*JAMA*) and *Pharmacy and Therapeutics* have published articles on the solid science behind the healing patterns that Eastern cultures have witnessed for millennia and that William O'Shaughnessy and other Western doctors have seen for nearly two centuries.

THE STORY OF HEMP CBD

Up to now, it's been impossible to tell the story of one hemp variety without the other: marijuana, hemp, and their components have been intertwined. From here on in, hemp and its component CBD will move into the limelight. It's time to discuss healing without the high.

In 1940, researcher Roger Adams and colleagues in the United States isolated a chemical compound from the cannabis plant that they called cannabidiol (CBD). A similar compound, tetrahydrocannabinol (THC), was identified in the United Kingdom by a group of chemists in 1942: H. J. Wollner, John Matchett, Joseph Levine, and S. Loewe. While THC had psychoactive properties, CBD did not. Little more research took place until 1960, when the Israeli chemist Dr. Raphael Mechoulam and his team discerned CBD's chemical structure.

CBD's chemical structure was barely different from THC's, but just enough to give it the non-high-inducing quality. This discovery set the stage for identifying

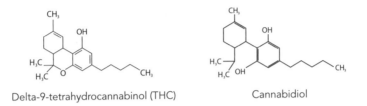

Delta-9-tetrahydrocannabinol (THC)   Cannabidiol

other compounds, called cannabinoids, in both marijuana and hemp and how they balance and heal the body. Over the next four decades, Dr. Mechoulam's lab learned that, by interacting with receptors throughout the body, THC, CBD, and other cannabinoids might calm nausea or epilepsy or boost mood and immunity, and so much more.

If such a miraculous treatment was percolating in such a highly respected researcher's lab, why did it take so long for CBD to become mainstream in the United States? Because for nearly a century, hemp in both forms had been blacklisted. Marijuana, though enjoyed in college dorms and beyond, remained on the U.S. government's Schedule 1 list of controlled—addictive and illegal—substances. Hemp, while rich with CBD and other non-psychoactive components and non-habit-forming, sat beside it. It would take advocacy by doctors, chemists, parents with sick children, and other experts—and some 60 years from Mechoulam's first discovery—for marijuana to become legal for medical use in 34 states and for hemp to have its day.

Modern public awareness of CBD as a healer remained relatively dormant until 2009, when a little girl with epilepsy helped launch it into the limelight. The parents of three-year-old Charlotte Figi, who could go barely an hour without a seizure, worked with hemp growers in Colorado to develop a CBD-THC mixture called Charlotte's Web. The product, which immediately calmed Charlotte, was made from the marijuana plant and had higher than a 0.3 percent dose of intoxicating THC. Still, it opened the door for CBD to be respected as a potential remedy and for researchers to work even harder to focus on CBD's values alone.

Late in 2018, for all states across the U.S., the Farm Bill legalized low-THC, CBD-rich hemp (see page 26). Once the source of rope, cloth, and seeds that promote shiny hair, the hemp plant's leaves, stem, and flowers are now being studied and tested by scientists to create remedies for some of Earth's most challenging conditions.

LET'S GET SPECIFIC: ALL ABOUT CBD

A miracle drug? We won't go quite that far, but let's definitely sit up and take notice. What exactly does CBD do? Which practices have been carried forward through time? And how can CBD be useful to you today as an alternative or addition to prescription drugs?

We'll take a closer look at its interaction with the body below, but the topline answer from scientists is this: CBD appears to play a role in regulating the transmission of chemical signals throughout the body. This healthy transmission helps keep our systems balanced and free from depression, memory loss, diabetes, heart disease, seizures, bone weakening, neurodegenerative diseases, and so much more.

CBD: The Plentiful Phytocannabinoid

Since Raphael Mechoulam's early work in 1960, scientists have discovered that CBD is one of more than 100 chemical compounds, called cannabinoids, found in the marijuana and hemp plants. Cannabinoids interact with a vital regulatory system in our body called the endocannabinoid system (ECS). To fuel this system, the body naturally makes its own cannabinoids, called endocannabinoids (*endo* is a prefix meaning "inside"). Plant cannabinoids, called phytocannabinoids, can be consumed to boost the ECS when it does not make enough endocannabinoids of its own.

Both marijuana and hemp happen to be rich in phytocannabinoids. In fact, they are the only plants known by scientists to *contain* phytocannabinoids. And one thing more: research shows that CBD is the most abundant of all phytocannabinoids.

Body Balancer: The Endocannabinoid System

To understand how vital the roles of endo- and phytocannabinoids are, it is important to comprehend the role of our endocannabinoid system. The ECS has two main jobs:

1. To keep the body in homeostasis, or functioning in a healthy, happy, balanced way. The ECS is a widespread network of receptors, endocannabinoids, and enzymes that regulates chemical messages sent between cells to balance such bodily functions as breathing, heartbeat, appetite, pain sensation, inflammation control, immune system function, memory, mood, and sleep.

2. To restore the body after it experiences internal or external stressors. The ECS interacts with the endocannabinoids it produces and with phytocannabinoids that come from the hemp plant. Together, these cannabinoids can help play a dramatic role in restoring balance to bodily systems upset by conditions such as injury or disease.

Not even a glimmer in our eye until a few decades ago, knowledge of the ECS began taking tangible shape in the 1990s through the continued research of Raphael Mechoulam. In the 30-year hiatus since determining the different chemical structures and effects of THC and CBD, he had been leading studies using these phytocannabinoids to treat seizures and other disorders.

By 1992 he'd determined that not only plants but also human bodies produce their own form of cannabinoids, or endocannabinoids. Further, he found that the body's endocannabinoids played a major part in the ECS balancing act, by interacting with its receptors and enzymes. Soon he and other researchers had an initial grasp of how such compounds—whether plant or human—react with the ECS, to keep it and the body humming or to pick it up when it falters. Their discoveries opened the door to exploring this wide-ranging and rich system with its enormous healing potential.

The Basic Idea: How the ECS Works

To keep the body in a balanced state of homeostasis, the ECS uses three main components to ensure smooth neurotransmission, or messaging between cells. These include:

CANNABINOID RECEPTORS, which are abundant throughout the body and attach to cell membranes to monitor the messages between cells and to keep bodily actions and systems running smoothly. For example, receptors in key parts of the brain control pain, motor activity, appetite, memory, and nausea while receptors in the greater body manage our digestive, reproductive, and immune systems.

ENDOCANNABINOIDS or fat-rich molecules that activate cannabinoid receptors and signal other systems to support the ECS when homeostasis is disrupted.

ENZYMES or catalysts that produce endocannabinoids to interact with receptors when the ECS is imbalanced.

There are six main cannabinoid receptors in our bodies and in CBD. The most important receptors are Cannabinoid-1 and -2 (or CB1 and CB2). When the body's homeostasis is threatened by injury or illness, cell messaging goes haywire. Then our body calls on receptors like CB1 and CB2, among others, as reinforcements. Four other receptors—5-HT1A, TRPV-1, GPR55, and GABA-A—address the ECS system's more specific needs (see sidebar on page 20).

Soon, endocannabinoids are on the scene. These fat-rich molecules rush to activate the receptors, causing a chemical reaction that gets cell messaging back on track. Endocannabinoid molecules also signal other systems to support the ECS during the crisis.

The endocannabinoid molecules have been produced on demand by the ECS enzymes. When the problem is fixed, the enzymes break those molecules down—and the system goes humming along again.

How efficiently the ECS functions and maintains homeostasis depends on a person's general health and diet, and on environmental stressors, genetics, and age. Perhaps your genetic coding points to the potential for ADHD, causing a natural blip in the ECS receptors' smooth cell messaging. Perhaps you have a high-stress lifestyle with a poor diet, which lowers enzyme activity and their production of endocannabinoids. Researchers in recent years have paired low endocannabinoid production with such conditions as seizure disorders, anxiety, depression, and menstrual pain, and with neurodegenerative disorders like Parkinson's disease and multiple sclerosis.

For these reasons, researchers starting with Mechoulam have looked to reinforce endocannabinoid production—and to boost the vital ECS—by supplementing it with the phytocannabinoids found in both hemp varieties. They've discovered that, like the body-produced endocannabinoids, plant-produced cannabinoids can help boost receptor activity and restore smooth messaging between cells to balance and heal the body. That means CBD—the most plentiful of all phytocannabinoids—is on the front lines of this exciting research.

Along with CBD, some 100 other phytocannabinoids help strengthen the ECS. Besides their cell-messaging support, phytocannabinoids bring other healing powers. Similar to flavonoids, another class of plant compounds, phytocannabinoids are rich in vitamins and minerals that deliver antioxidant, anti-inflammatory, and relaxation effects. They also contain terpenes, some 15 aromatic oils also found in such healing herbs as lavender, black pepper, and hops. They give plants their scent and flavor but also interact with other plant compounds, like phytocannabinoids, to heal. They contribute to muscle relaxation, pain and inflammation control, bacteria resistance, memory function, mood balance, cancer protection, and so much more.

In healthy people, scientists are finding that regular use of phytocannabinoid supplements may well keep in check chronic inflammation, which prompts autoimmune and degenerative disorders, and free radical buildup, which leads to cell damage, aging, memory loss, and disease.

Recent findings show that CBD in particular helps maintain health and rebalance upset systems by building the endocannabinoid supply and increasing endocannabinoid-receptor interaction. That is, it helps a person maintain "endocannabinoid tone."

CBD, maintains neurologist Dr. Ethan Russo, a leader in ECS research, "on its own has many properties that THC doesn't—as an anti-anxiety agent, as an anti-psychotic, and doing all this without producing intoxication." For much of its history, CBD has been considered more or less a "helpmate" to the powerful phytocannabinoid THC. At the 2018 Cannabis Conference in Vermont, one

KNOW YOUR CANNABINOID RECEPTORS

CB1 receptors populate the brain and the central nervous system and spread throughout the body's cells, concentrating in organs, glands, tissues, and systems.

CB2 receptors overlap with the CB1 receptors mainly in parts of the body outside the brain; they concentrate in white blood cells, and they play a key role in protecting the immune system.

5-HT1A receptors, like CB1, situate in the brain and help regulate appetite, pain, sleep, and mood, with the help of the neurotransmitter serotonin, known for triggering feelings of happiness.

TRPV-1 receptors, like CB2, are mainly found in the body outside the central nervous system. TRPV-1 helps keep pain and inflammation in check and plays a role in moderating body temperature.

GPR55 receptors help regulate blood pressure and maintain bone density, guarding against osteoporosis, hypertension, and other disease. They position specifically in the brain's cerebellum and in osteoblasts, or bone-building cells.

GABA-A receptors lie in the central nervous system. Research reveals that this receptor likely helps regulate anxiety, and when activated by the hemp CBD phytocannabinoid, it protects against convulsions and may help keep seizures in check.

producer said,, "We consider CBD the portal—getting you just so far toward the healing process, but then THC takes over as the true healer." As more research is being done, however, CBD is quickly becoming known as a healer in its own right. Says Russo, "Clearly, this is a substance that has a lot to offer on many levels."

Dr. Christopher Shade, a former organic farmer turned environmental metals chemist, has spent much of his life determining how to detoxify the human body from metals we consume daily through our environment—as we eat, sleep, and breathe. His and other chemists' studies have shown how CBD—well apart from THC—takes specialized pathways through the ECS to shore up our nervous, immune, and peripheral body systems. It can play a major role not only in detoxing the body, but also in controlling inflammation, enhancing mood, blocking disease, and more.

Mechoulam's discovery of the endocannabinoid system set us on the path to gaining insight into how CBD works with the body's ECS and why it can be effective for treating many different illnesses and conditions. The rest of the book will explore these conditions and how they respond to CBD.

THE INTEGRATIVE ECS

The degree to which a CBD supplement benefits the ECS will depend on how well it interacts with this system. That means keeping the ECS in tip-top shape. Doing that requires what we might call a "team effort." For optimal production of endocannabinoids and uptake of phytocannabinoids, you need to keep your system humming through other means as well.

An integrative approach is key, based on these pillars:

BALANCED DIET: That means foods balanced in omega-6 and omega-3 fatty acids, which support endocannabinoid production. Flaxseed, hemp seed oil, and nuts contain both; corn, sunflower, and soybean oils contain omega-6; and avocado, green leafy vegetables, and cold-water, high-fat fish like salmon are rich in omega-3. The balance between these acids is key, with the most beneficial ratio being from 1:1 to 5:1 omega-6 to omega-3. Overconsumption of vegetable oils, especially from processed foods, can blow the omega-6

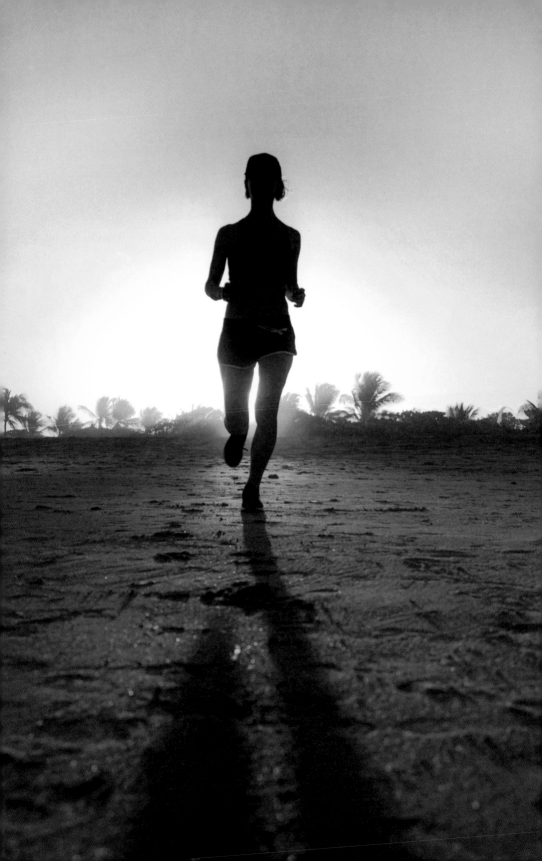

level out of the water—to a ratio of 16:1 or higher. Here's the bottom line: the higher the omega-6 part of the ratio, the lower the production of endocannabinoids, the higher the inability to maintain homeostasis, and the higher the propensity to develop diabetes, heart conditions, and other disease.

Another dietary plus comes from probiotic bacteria in fermented foods such as yogurt and sauerkraut. Studies show that probiotics increase the responsiveness of cannabinoid receptors in the intestines and promote gut homeostasis.

EXERCISE: This mighty medicine has been hailed as the 20th-century wonder drug because that's when scientists began realizing its extraordinary capacity to maintain wellness and to heal. How does it play with the ECS? Animal and human studies underscore its positive effects: In animals, sustained movement has been seen to increase both cannabinoid receptors in the brain and their interaction with endocannabinoids. In humans, running, swimming, biking, and other quickstepping exercise shows increased endocannabinoid levels in the blood—a possible explanation (besides the endorphins theory) behind the euphoria we sometimes label "runner's high."

SLEEP: Quality sleep is our natural reset button. While scientists don't fully understand why we need to sleep, they know that it makes us more alert and able to learn and socialize; it wards off inflammation and pain; it helps us manage stress; it allows us to stay physically agile; and it helps us control weight—all actions that are also regulated by a healthy ECS. Scientists have found that in the healthy ECS, certain endocannabinoids increase in number at night and that certain receptors are more responsive to them. These work together to promote the optimal amount of sleep—between seven and eight hours for adults. Sleep in turn nourishes the ECS—a symbiosis we can all live with.

STRESS MANAGEMENT: While we all need and thrive on certain amounts of stress—to keep life interesting and to move our worlds forward—a state of chronic stress can challenge your health and even shorten your life. Over time, coping mechanisms such as becoming a workaholic, drinking, lying awake to plan or worry, and missing meals or overindulging all contribute to heightened loss of well-being. A 2016 NIH study showed that chronic stress decreases the production of both ECS receptors and endocannabinoids, not only lowering the ability to fight inflammation and protect immune function but also setting the stage for conditions such as anxiety, chronic pain, memory loss, depression, and post-traumatic stress. So reevaluating your 18-hour, full-speed-ahead day—and calming down—is a priority.

SPIRITUALITY: You may not believe in a specific higher being, but there appears to be benefit in recognizing that there is a greater, all-encompassing power, that we are not responsible for everything, and that we can basically "hand over" our fears and hopes and health concerns, to be nourished by a universal energy. For centuries, traditional healers have prescribed yoga, meditation, acupuncture, qigong (a Chinese relaxation exercise related to tai chi), fasting, chanting, and limpias (a Mexican spiritual cleansing). And there is prayer—often considered a Western concept. Through time, scientists have observed, these activities evoke a "relaxation response," promoting health both mental and physical. Experts believe that such practices help the ECS remain balanced, warding off stress and the diseases it triggers.

SOCIALIZATION: As with the premise for spirituality, we all need to know that we are not alone in our immediate worlds. Friendship, love, and lasting relationships—with a friend, a lover, a spouse, a child, a parent or grandparent, a person in need, a pet—are the foundations for meaning in life and for joy. More than that, they are the basis for health and longevity. Through time, studies show that giving and receiving in a deep social attachment increases a chemical called oxytocin, which in turn reinforces trust and empathy and decreases stress, anxiety, depression, pain, and inflammation while encouraging optimal heart rate. All point to helping the ECS maintain balance.

These pillars play a vital role in supporting healing from the common ailments and conditions you'll read about in Chapter 3. While that chapter focuses on how CBD strengthens the ECS to promote healing, it's important to recognize that these pillars, in addition to CBD, can help promote healing and prosperity.

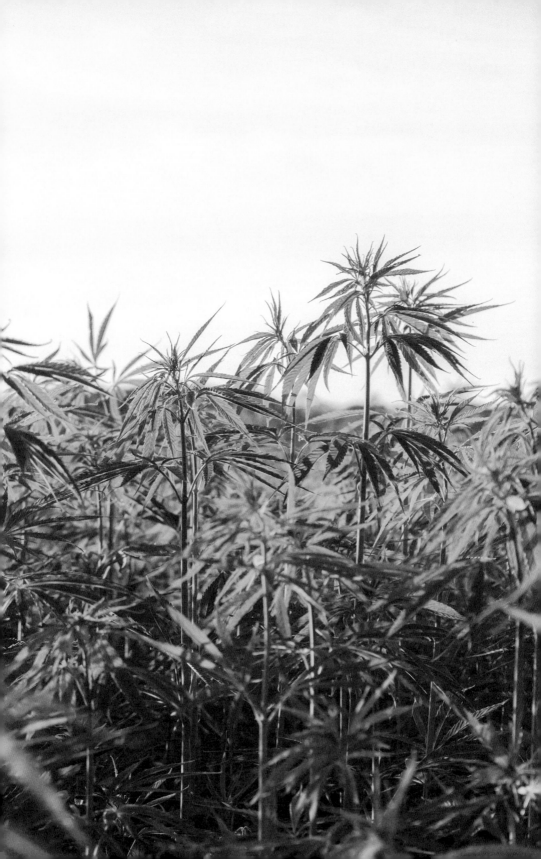

THE SKINNY ON CBD: FAQS

Can CBD Ever Make Me High?

No . . . and yes. CBD acts on different pathways through the body's ECS than does THC, so you cannot become intoxicated using it alone. However, the hemp plant from which CBD is extracted does contain low levels of THC. So if you're ingesting supplements that contain large concentrations of CBD extract, it's possible that they have enough THC to make you high. You could also experience intoxication if the particular hemp plant used for extraction has had an accidental infusion of THC because a THC-rich cannabis plant was growing nearby or the two were processed at the same plant. That's why relying on a trusted manufacturing source that tests both CBD and THC levels during supplement production is key. Guidance from a CBD-savvy health care professional about the safest product to purchase is also important. These precautions are a must. If you don't do your work up front, you may pay the price with an unwanted intoxicating experience or by failing a drug test.

What's the Federal Regulation?

All cannabis plants, whether CBD-rich hemp or THC-rich marijuana, remain under the cannabis umbrella on the Schedule 1 list of illegal substances in the Controlled Substances Act (CSA) of 1970. While both are becoming more accepted as healers, in many states it has long been illegal to grow any hemp or marijuana plant unless you've been certified and approved to use it for research or medical needs. Products with THC must be bought with a medical prescription. CBD-based products with no trace of THC can be bought over the counter.

In the meantime, it's important to note that since 2003, the United States Department of Health and Human Services (USDHH) has held Patent No. 6,630,507, stating that cannabinoids—which would include CBD, THC, and the other 100 compounds in hemp and marijuana plants—have been found to have antioxidant properties and to aid inflammatory and autoimmune diseases, brain recovery from stroke, epilepsy, and neurodegenerative diseases such as Parkinson's, Alzheimer's, and HIV dementia.

In 2014, Congress passed the Agricultural Act, known as the Farm Bill, permitting pilot crops of hemp to be grown, processed, and marketed as long as the percentage of THC is under 0.3 percent—and as long as growers and producers are properly licensed. The 2018 Farm Bill expands on the 2014 bill, allowing broader hemp cultivation, not just for pilot programs. It also lifts restrictions on the sale, transport, and possession of hemp-derived products.

In addition, as of June of 2018, the product Epidiolex—which uses CBD derived from marijuana but without THC—has been approved by the FDA as a treatment for certain forms of extreme epilepsy. Results have shown a drop in monthly seizures as great as 37 percent.

This is good news for you. It means that the U.S. government is aware of the healing powers of both THC and CBD and that it's making promising steps toward allowing their use in widely available medicines. It also means that the government is instituting safety standards. While all CBD and other hemp products should go through a careful vetting process to allow for safe usage, that is not always the case. It's true that careful manufacturers are making life-changing products, but others are creating cheap products for fast money—and you need to know the difference. Some call the current atmosphere "the Wild West." The good news is that CBD appears to be a gold mine waiting to deliver. In the next pages we'll guide you on how to look carefully at CBD's effects on different conditions and how you can buy optimal, safe products.

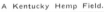
A Kentucky Hemp Field.

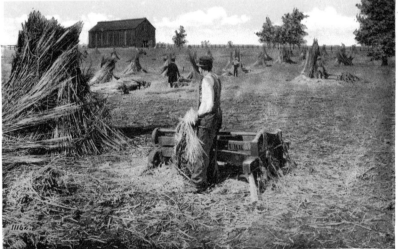

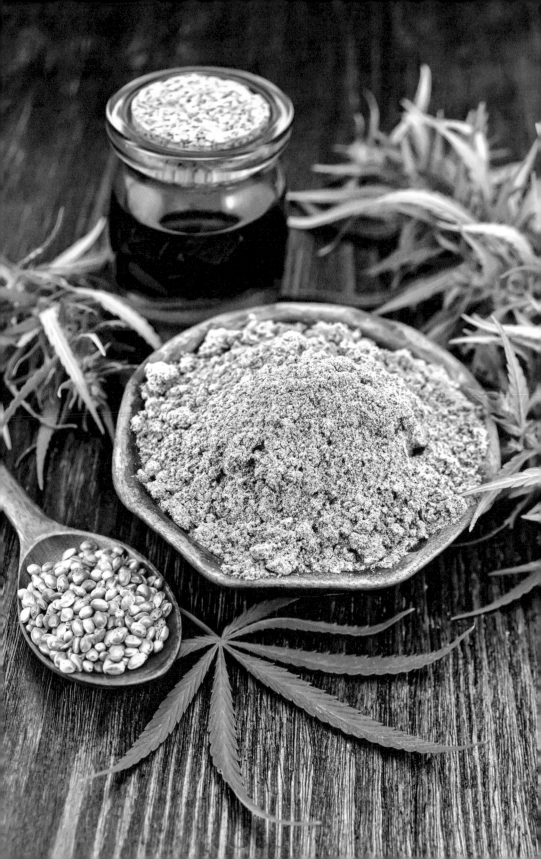

PART TWO

Choosing CBD

HOW DO YOU KNOW IF CBD IS FOR YOU?

Before adding CBD to your wellness routine, always talk to a trusted health care provider, especially one who understands the ins and outs of hemp CBD. You will also need to do the following:

KNOW YOUR STUFF. Read up and develop an understanding of your condition and of how CBD has been shown to affect it in a positive way. For additional materials beyond this book, check out the Further Reading section on page 213. After doing some further research, speak with your health care professionals about possible supplementation with CBD. In this chapter, you'll learn about extraction methods; product types; how to read a product label with its supplement fact panel for key elements and for harmful ones; and dosage levels. For more information on reading labels, see page 51.

STAY CURRENT. Keep an updated and complete list of your allergies, conditions, and prescriptions and their side effects. Patients with chronic conditions who are taking prescription drugs will always have to watch for potential interactions with CBD and other cannabinoid-rich medicines.

BE HONEST WITH YOURSELF. Consider your lifestyle and your willingness to welcome CBD into your wellness regimen. Will your finances support it? Are you prepared to put up with a trial period to assess interactions with your other medications? Will you commit to using it for the purposes you need, in the correct dosages?

STAY WATCHFUL. While following the guidelines determined with your health care professional, it can also be helpful to monitor your reaction to any product you take. Consider keeping a daily journal and report any side effects or noticeable drug interactions, such as dizziness or weakness. Then work with the professional to balance your dosage. "It's important to report the positive changes, too," says Deanna Gabriel Vierck, "such as better sleep, calmer mood, or relaxed pain. As a practitioner, it's amazing to me how easily we forget our degree of suffering once it has passed. Our brains are designed to do this so we can move beyond a challenge."

Try tracking your own CBD healing progress by filling in the checklist on the following pages. In it, you'll rate your symptoms before and during the use of a new product to determine how it may be helping or hindering.

TRACKING CBD SUPPLEMENT EFFECTS

Please plan to fill this out prior to taking a CBD supplement for the first time. (We suggest photocopying this or scanning it into your computer for future use.) Rate each experience based on what is true for you before using CBD. Then review the information after taking the supplement for two to four weeks. Ideally, you'll fill out this chart again after two weeks using the supplement, and again after four weeks. Use the number ranges at the top of the chart to indicate changes in the way you feel. You are encouraged to record any additional thoughts or observations in the space provided at the end of the chart.

	Before	2 weeks after	4 weeks after
Name:			
Date:			

0   never have the symptom

1–2   rarely have the symptom

3–4   occasional symptom, effect not severe

5–6   occasional symptom, effect severe

7–8   frequent symptom, effect not severe

9–10   frequent symptom, effect severe

	Before	2 weeks after	4 weeks after
Digestion			
Belching or passing gas			
Bloated feeling			
Constipation			
Diarrhea			
Heartburn			
Nausea or vomiting			
Stomach pains or cramps			
Other			
Ears			
Earaches, ear infections			
Drainage from ear			
Itchy ears			
Fullness of ears			
Ringing in ears, hearing loss			
Other			

	Before	2 weeks after	4 weeks after
Emotions			
Aggressiveness			
Anger/Irritability			
Anxiety/Fears			
Depression			
Mood swings			
Other			
Energy and Activity			
Apathy/lethargy			
Fatigue/sluggishness			
Hyperactivity			
Restlessness			
Eyes			
Blurred vision			
Dark circles around eyes			
Spots before eyes			
Swollen or sticky eyelids			
Watery or itchy			
Other			
Head			
Dizziness			
Drowsiness			
Insomnia			
Faintness			
Other			

	Before	2 weeks after	4 weeks after
Heart			
Chest pain			
Irregular heartbeat			
Pounding or rapid heartbeat			
Other			
Joints and Muscles			
Arthritis			
Numbness			
Pains or aches in joints			
Pains or aches in muscles			
Swelling in hands or feet			
Weakness			
Other			
Lungs			
Asthma/bronchitis			
Chest congestion			
Difficulty breathing			
Shortness of breath			
Nose			
Excessive mucus			
Hay fever			
Sinus problems			
Sneezing attacks			
Stuffy nose, smell altered			
Other			

	Before	2 weeks after	4 weeks after
Mind			
Difficulty making decisions			
Learning disabilities			
Poor comprehension			
Poor concentration			
Poor physical coordination			
Poor memory			
Stuttering			
Other			
Mouth and Throat			
Canker sores			
Chronic coughing			
Dry or itching in mouth			
Frequent throat-clearing			
Frequent sore throat			
Hoarseness			
Metallic taste			
Other			
Skin			
Acne			
Dandruff			
Excessive sweating			
Change in color			
Flushing or hot flashes			
Hives, rash, or dry skin			
Thin hair			
Other			

	Before	2 weeks after	4 weeks after
Weight			
Present weight _____lbs.			
Binge eating/drinking			
Crave certain foods? Which ones?			
Water retention			
Other			
Frequent illness			
Frequent urination			
Genital itch or discharge			
Anything Else?			

KNOW CBD EXTRACTION FOR SAFE USE

Manufacturers use different extraction methods to draw CBD out of the plant for addition to the many products on the market. It's important to know these methods and to look for them on the product labels; each has pros and cons you'll want to consider.

Cold Pressing

This method is used for hemp seeds only. Simply, the hemp seeds are placed in a press, which squeezes the oil out of the seeds. If you see the term "cold pressed," pause and consider: you are buying a hemp seed oil—which will be packed with omega-6 and omega-3 nutrients. These support healthy skin, hair, and more. But you won't be buying a hemp CBD oil, which has ECS interaction and therefore more advanced healing effects.

Carbon Dioxide (CO_2) Extraction Method

This is usually considered the safest method—and the most beneficial for the environment. It's also time-tested: it's the standard method for removing caffeine from coffee and essential oils from herbs such as lavender and rosemary. To extract the CBD oil from the hemp plant, the plant is placed in an extraction vessel along with CO_2. Then experts apply very high pressure and very low temperatures to allow the CO_2 to pull the CBD from the plant. The final product is safe, pure, and potent for medicinal purposes. It retains other healing components of the hemp—for the entourage effect (see page 50)—while removing chlorophyll and other unwanted residuals. Then the CO_2 is recycled back into the atmosphere. Two slightly different versions of the method are called subcritical (low temperature throughout the process) or supercritical (high temperature that is then lowered)—but the result is the same. The method requires intricate, expensive equipment and experts who know how to use it. You'll pay a top price for it—but health care professionals hold that the pure product is worth it.

Ethanol Extraction

Ethanol is another name for alcohol. In this method, the hemp plant is submerged in high-grade ethanol. The mixture in turn goes into separation equipment that aids in drawing out medicinal CBD oil, along with other beneficial plant components, including terpenes and flavonoids. While this method yields an end product similar to the CO_2-extracted product, in some cases it may use plant material that is not top grade and may leave in toxic residuals. For this method, testing by a third-party lab is recommended. The ethanol extract is also sometimes termed a tincture (see page 43) and is often the first step toward creating an isolate (as in "isolation"). (See Isolate Powders, page 41.)

Olive Oil Extraction

This simple method places the hemp plant in olive oil and allows the oil to leach out the CBD component. You'll use the oil itself—which retains both CBD and other healthful components from the hemp plant—as the supplement. This requires no special equipment, and people who have access to the hemp plant often make their own home remedies. One downside is that contaminants can make their way in, turning the oil rancid more quickly than manufactured products. Another downside is that over time the oil may go rancid before the CBD itself does. Once bought or made, it must be stored in a cool, dark place, at less than 77°F. Generally, an oil-based product stored properly will remain fresh from a few months to a year. When purchasing, look for the label's expiration date.

KNOW CBD DELIVERY SYSTEMS

Depending on your need, CBD can be taken in a variety of ways: ingested as a capsule or drop, applied topically as a salve, or inhaled as a vapor. Each form and individual product has a different potential absorption level. The delivery system can impact the quick, efficient, and lasting effect of CBD. For every product, you must learn to read the labels carefully, both for dosage guidance and to ensure it has no harmful elements such as artificial colors or flavors, corn syrup, or unwanted plant residuals, like chlorophyll. Find out more about label reading and dosage on pages 51 and 57. And always coordinate with your health care professional before using any of these products.

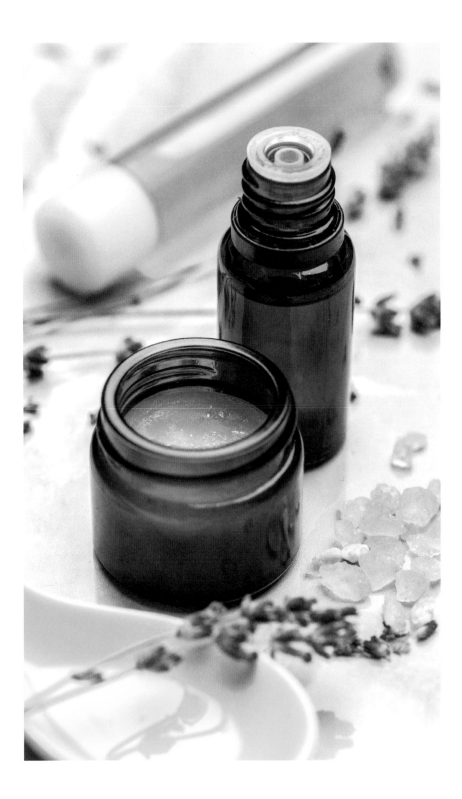

Ingested

CAPSULES

Usually in the form of gel caps, this delivery system may be the easiest way to begin taking hemp CBD. You'll usually find soft gels made of concentrated oil or powder covered by a gelatin capsule. They come in a range of sizes and strengths, so you'll need to carefully read the label and use as directed.

WHY IT MAY WORK FOR YOU: Capsules offer effectiveness over a long period of time, especially if it's important to keep CBD levels consistent in your body. This product is often recommended for ongoing conditions, such as arthritis pain or asthma.

CONCERNS: There may be a significant delay in experiencing relief. With this delivery system, it takes a while for the digestive system to break down the capsules so that the CBD can circulate into the bloodstream. Also, dosage can be tricky, both because of the slower absorption time and because the dosage is set—you can't easily adjust it as you can with liquid dispensed through a dropper or pump. Finally, while most people ingest these capsules easily, some may experience an upset stomach if the powder inside contains raw plant material. Those who frequently experience bloating, diarrhea, constipation, or other gastrointestinal upsets may have a challenging time digesting and absorbing capsules.

EDIBLES: FOODS, BEVERAGES, CANDY, AND LOZENGES

Gummies, chocolate bars, popcorn, tea. Delicious and easy to ingest, these products are generally made using CBD-infused oils or by adding drops of tinctures or measures of isolate powders from one of the extractions on pages 36–37. While foods, beverages, candies, and lozenges can be soothing for certain ailments such as cough or sore throat, or for delivering a dose of well-being, they are weaker than concentrated drops or pills and don't usually deliver healing over a long period of time. That said, the recipes beginning on page 131 combine hemp CBD supplements with other healing components, such as herbs and nutrient-dense foods. Simple drinks and food are a great way to start using CBD and to begin feeling its healing effects. Here is a sampling of the different drinkable and edible products available on the market.

Herbal teas and other beverages: Imagine a steaming, aromatic cup of tea that delivers the healing powers of CBD—heavenly. Teas made from infusions (steeped leaves and flowers) or diffusions (roots and other parts boiled, then steeped) of nutrient-rich, healing herbs such as echinacea, red clover, or ginger are a great place to start. Because buying hemp leaf is generally illegal unless it's for research purposes, it is best to make a tea from other healing herbs, and then add the CBD drops. A dropper or more of CBD tincture, depending on type and strength, enhances the herbal tea's natural healing powers. Drops can also be added to water, juice, hot chocolate, tea and coffee lattes, and more. Just remember that CBD mixed into any drink is diluted and not as immediately effective as taken alone. Recent packaged products include teas that are a blend of herbs, infused with CBD; cold teas and juices are also available. And the near future may bring CBD beer, too. As always, check the labels for the content and dosage of CBD.

Lozenges and gum: Often made with CBD isolates that work efficiently, the uptake here is quick as you chew or suck: the mucous membranes under the tongue absorb the medicine into your system in as little as 20 minutes, soothing your sore or itchy throat, calming a cough, or helping relieve general inflammation associated with colds and flu. It is important to note that it has not been documented to unblock nasal passages. Check labels for the amount of CBD in each individual piece and look for sugar-free versions, too.

Foods: From salad dressing and pesto (check out the one on page 178) to gummies and carob-chip energy balls, making recipes is a great way to begin experimenting with and understanding CBD. For many recipes you can use drops of CBD tincture, concentrate, or isolate. It's important to always add it at the end of the cooking process because heat destroys its therapeutic effect. Because food needs to process through the digestive system in order to deliver its goods, the CBD uptake is much slower than with other delivery methods—perhaps one to three hours. For that reason, if you're not feeling the effects after 20 minutes, be patient and let it take hold. (That is, don't immediately eat another double fudge brownie if the dosage calls for just one!)

WHY IT MAY WORK FOR YOU: Especially for the beginner, a number of products are available that will make uptake easy as well as beneficial. Gummies, apple cider vinegar, and chocolate bars are among the choices. For those who have trouble swallowing capsules or who feel uncomfortable dropping a quick-acting product under their tongue, a food, beverage, or candy is a moderating delivery system.

CONCERNS: It's easy to overindulge if the CBD doesn't seem to be acting immediately. Overconsumption won't hurt you, but if the CBD hasn't been adequately refined to separate out THC or soil toxins, too much can lead to unwanted drowsiness.

ISOLATE POWDERS

This fine white crystalline powder is an even purer form of hemp CBD than the sublingual concentrate (see the following page). To make it, CBD oil is pulled from the hemp plant via the CO_2 extraction method and then refined to to a powder that contains 99 percent pure CBD. Any oils, fatty acids, waxes, chlorophyll, and other plant components that remain in the concentrated CBD oil have been removed. The CBD has been "isolated" out through a chemical process. This powder dissolves easily and can be used to make many products.

WHY IT MAY WORK FOR YOU: This concentrate has focused healing properties of CBD, with hugely efficient absorption into the body through the bloodstream. That makes it a strong and immediate remedy for acute pain, nausea, menstrual cramps, or other specific ailments.

CONCERNS: This product is missing key plant compounds, like other cannabinoids, terpenes, and flavonoids, that add to the entourage effect (page 50). Additionally, with an isolate, once the absorption level is reached, the body cannot absorb any more. This keeps it from being a useful remedy for long-term chronic conditions.

NANO-LIPOSOMAL OILS

Sometimes called CBD water, this product begins as CBD extracted through the CO_2 or ethanol extraction methods explained earlier. An additional process called nano-liposomal (*nano* meaning "small" and *liposomal* meaning "fat-injected") makes the CBD molecules extremely minute and then encloses them in a layer of lipid, or fat. The molecules' tiny size and the absorption-aiding fat layer promote efficient uptake into the central nervous and lymphatic system, a network of tissues and organs in the vascular and immune system that help rid the body of toxins. This concentrated and efficient delivery system generally requires a lower dosage than other forms of CBD.

WHY IT MAY WORK FOR YOU: A smaller CBD dosage and immediate uptake, as little as 30 seconds, may be more desirable for your condition, especially in acute situations such as migraine or injury pain, menstrual cramps, and nausea.

CONCERNS: The nano-liposomal formula is in an early stage of development and use. One school of thought is that while the small molecules appear to improve efficient CBD uptake, impurities, such as fungus or trace metals, may creep into the product and may also be delivered efficiently. Generally, experts are not seeing this happen. Still, read the label for the manufacturer's statement of purity.

SUBLINGUAL CONCENTRATES

These are without a doubt the fastest delivery system for CBD. Concentrates are simply this: the pure hemp CBD oil extracted from the hemp plant via the CO_2 extraction method. While it contains other plant materials, such as valuable fatty acids, it is not combined with other ingredients, such as alcohol or oil. For this product, the label will state that there are no other ingredients. Dosage is generally a tiny drop, often described as equivalent in size to a grain of rice.

WHY IT MAY WORK FOR YOU: This product is no-fuss, no-mix. It simply requires understanding of the dosage size and carefully administering the tiny amount under the tongue. Patients with ongoing medical conditions often prefer this for its quick uptake, which can be under a minute, and it can last for six to eight hours.

CONCERNS: This extremely concentrated product must be taken carefully so that only the recommended dose, not more, is ingested. Also, be sure to read the label carefully to ensure that the oil is extracted from the hemp plant, since this method is also used for CBD extracted from the marijuana plant.

SUBLINGUAL SPRAYS AND DROPS

Among all delivery systems, sprays and drops have the lowest amount of CBD per serving. That said, they can also be the fastest and most effective forms of CBD supplementation because of their immediate uptake and significantly higher absorption rate. While you can purchase sublingual sprays or drops as pure CBD extracts, many come mixed with a delivery substance like coconut oil and in flavors including peppermint, mango, lemon, and strawberry. To use such a product, you'll follow the directions to spray or drop it under your tongue. Here the blood vessels aid in quick uptake, as little as 30 seconds, and circulation through your system. This is faster than swallowing and digesting a pill.

WHY IT MAY WORK FOR YOU: Because of the low concentration, it is often recommended for beginners. Its quick uptake makes it a go-to calming remedy for nausea and anxiety.

CONCERNS: These are easy products to make, so beware of homemade recipes. They can contain bacteria and mold if they've not been made under pristine conditions. As with all CBD products, it is key to read the label to be sure of the contents and the instructions.

TINCTURES AND GLYCERITES

A tincture is a time-honored delivery system for herbal medicines: an herb is fully soaked in alcohol for days, weeks, or sometimes months. Over time the liquid extracts the active, healing ingredients from the herb, in this case from the hemp plant. The resulting alcohol tincture is a concentrated healer. Today, the mechanical ethanol extraction process explained on page 37 is usually used to make alcohol tinctures. Alcohol tinctures absorb most quickly into the bloodstream—but they're very strong. Combining them with either glycerin or oil delivers the tinctures' healing properties while diluting the alcohol's potent effect. Most CBD tinctures you'll find on the market are oil-based. Some newer products use all three solvents—alcohol, glycerin, and oil—to create a multi-solvent tincture.

Alcohol: Tinctures made with 190 proof, pure alcohol work most efficiently. This strong tincture cannot be dropped directly on or under the tongue, since it will burn sensitive membrane. But it can be added into drinks or foods for an uptake in about 30–60 minutes. Effects generally last six to eight hours. Directions on the label may recommend repeating the dosage several times in a day, depending on a person's need and condition.

Oil: It's the most common CBD supplement form on the market—basically an alcohol (ethanol)-based or CO_2 extraction diluted in a carrier oil such as coconut or olive. Drops can be put on or under the tongue for optimal uptake, up to about 75 minutes. It easily blends into soft foods like yogurt, applesauce, and smoothies; but it separates out of juice, water, and tea, so is not recommended in those drinks. The effect can last six to eight hours.

Glycerite: This is the name for a tincture that uses an ethanol- or alcohol-based or CO_2 extraction diluted in glycerin: a sweet-tasting, colorless liquid with a syrupy consistency that's drawn from lipids or fats, usually from the palm, soy, or coconut plant. A glycerite is not harsh in flavor, and it can be added to food and drink products. It can also be dropped on the tongue or under it for the quickest uptake—as little as 30 seconds, and up to two minutes. Again, the effect can last six to eight hours.

Multi-solvent: Some recent supplements combine all of the above tincture types into one powerhouse product, with quick uptake of as little as 30 seconds, with each type delivering its own benefit.

You may have made your own echinacea herbal tincture to treat colds, but making your own hemp CBD tincture is not so easy. A legal permit is required to grow and purchase the hemp plant for research only. In this book we recommend using ready-made tinctures you can purchase from a reputable source for recipes and in your wellness routine.

Tinctures usually come in small droppered glass bottles that often hold about an ounce of liquid. The glass is dark to protect the active ingredients from the dilution effect of light. The dropper aids in consistent and accurate dosing, with each dropperful delivering about 30 drops—that's 1 milliliter or ¼ teaspoon. Each product will differ slightly in potency and uptake, so the bottle's label gives guidelines for the optimal number of drops to use daily for that product (see Dosage Guidelines, page 54).

WHY IT MAY WORK FOR YOU: The concentration of healing plant compounds extracted through tinctures is generally very effective, with easy usage; uptake that can be as little as 30 seconds depending on the solvent used; and lasting effect, especially for chronic conditions that require ongoing usage.

CONCERNS: A straight alcohol tincture is strong: it can taste bitter and burn sensitive membrane if dropped directly on or under the tongue. For safe uptake, dilute it in any of a variety of liquids, from cranberry juice to water, or mix it in soft foods, such as applesauce or yogurt. That said, the alcohol tinctures diluted in oil or glycerin can be taken alone. For all tinctures, follow dosing recommendations carefully, starting low and building up to the highest dose, according to directions from your health care professional.

Topicals

PATCHES AND STRIPS

A CBD patch is a device for delivering CBD over a period of time—perhaps six to ten hours. Unlike topical lotions and salves, which address a concentrated area of irritation or infection on or near the top layer of skin, the CBD patch is usually transdermal. It is made by one of the CBD extraction methods above, mixed with a carrier or essential oil or other healing product, and put into a patch. While applied to the outer layer of skin, its CBD elements filter down through all seven skin layers to enter the bloodstream. It then spreads throughout the body to bring relief to the ailment. If you need a smaller amount of CBD, cut the patch into a smaller piece.

WHY IT MAY WORK FOR YOU: An animal study using the transdermal delivery system in several U.S. medical centers was published in the 2016 *European Journal of Pain*. It showed significant decrease in joint swelling and pain and projected its potential future use as a treatment for the some 50 million Americans suffering from various forms of arthritis.

CONCERNS: This is highly potent, and you must start slowly to ensure that you give yourself the optimal dosage. As always, be sure to consult a health care provider before starting this treatment.

Topical applications made by adding one of the CBD extractions above to a carrier salve, lotion, or oil are the least invasive of CBD products. They are used to treat conditions at the skin surface, such as psoriasis, eczema, and poison ivy. They also moderately soothe joint and arthritis pain and muscle soreness, especially when massaged gently into the skin and combined with essential oils, which aid absorption. Even more potent topical applications that sink through every layer of skin and deep into the bloodstream are called transdermal applications. (See Patches and Strips on page 45.)

WHY IT MAY WORK FOR YOU: Such topicals are immediately soothing for rashes and other skin conditions such as psoriasis and eczema. Thicker topicals may be combined with herbal lotions or oils for easier, more general application and for an additional healing boost, depending on the nature of the herb. A topical containing nano-liposomal oil, which is rich in healing lipids, or fats, is especially soothing to troubled skin. All topicals can soothe inflamed muscles and joints as well.

CONCERNS: For some people, topicals do not feel as if they're working right away, and they are abandoned. Be patient. Many people report that usage over time brings rewards.

Inhaled

VAPORS

Through vaporization, CBD's healing elements are released into the air unaccompanied by the toxic ones brought forth through smoking. To vaporize, heat drops of CBD to just below the combustion point, usually in a concentrate vaporizer or an e-liquid vaporizer. The concentrate version vaporizes pure CBD concentrates—CBD with no additional ingredients. Efficient delivery takes place through a pre-filled cartridge put into a vaporizer pen, which looks like a writing pen or permanent marker. Concentrates may come in flavors, including lemon, strawberry, and butterscotch. The e-liquid version is also available as a vape pen with a cartridge, but this method delivers CBD accompanied by other ingredients;

therefore it is less recommended, because it may release toxins when heated. Always read the label to know the ingredients.

WHY IT MAY WORK FOR YOU: By offering some of the satisfying effects of smoking without the harmful by-products, vaporizers have been found to help smokers shake nicotine addiction. Other successful uses have been for spasms, nausea, and vomiting.

CONCERNS: A report in the *New England Journal of Medicine* in 2015 spells out the toxins that appear through vaporizing, including formaldehyde. Additionally, the e-liquid version may contain unwanted components, such as propylene glycol, which releases carcinogens when heated. Toxic tobacco vaping episodes in 2019 opened the door for concerns for all forms fo vaping.

HOW TO CHOOSE A CBD PRODUCT

Know the Origin

Two main plants are used for extracting CBD. Get to know their pros and cons.

INDUSTRIAL HEMP

This plant, used traditionally for rope and cloth, has the minimally required 0.3 percent THC content to make it legal in the United States. It is a rich source of hemp seed used in hemp seed oil products. This particular plant doesn't have the same kind of flowering parts or the resin covering its stalk and leaves, which hold THC. Instead, its tall stalk is the go-to for CBD extract. It takes many stalks to make a little CBD, but as we're finding out, the product is worth it. CBD made from hemp is legal for purchase in all states since the Farm Bill passed in December 2018.

MEDICAL MARIJUANA

This book advises using the non-intoxicating hemp CBD, but you do need to know about medical marijuana to understand the CBD landscape. It's the traditional marijuana plant, whose products are made from the resin-rich leaves, stem, and flowers, which hold high levels of THC, CBD, and all the cannabinoids and nutrients. To make products from the medical marijuana plant, scientists extract THC to different levels, including to the lowest legal level of 0.3 percent or less. However, the final product is still considered a marijuana product. You can buy medical marijuana products in a dispensary in states where marijuana is legal. In states where recreational marijuana is illegal, you need to have a special medical license to purchase these products. And you can't have them shipped or taken by plane or car from legal to illegal states.

THE GRAY AREA: THERAPEUTIC HEMP

Under the umbrella of medical marijuana is a plant that is being cultivated from the marijuana plant to be largely void of THC while rich in CBD. It's been developed by growers federally approved to cultivate medical marijuana. To create the new plant, experts removed all resins but the minimally allowed 0.3 percent THC from the marijuana plant. By staying within this legal limit, they found they could reclassify their plants as hemp—and it's proving to be a step in the right direction. Many experts say that the CBD from this plant, along with other beneficial cannabinoids and terpenes, is richer and more potent—and its extracts more effective—than the CBD from industrial hemp. But it is important to note that therapeutic hemp is not openly approved for making legal hemp CBD products in the United States.

Know the Source

Industrial hemp has been grown for centuries around the world, in every environment and type of soil. Like any plant, hemp is a bioaccumulater: it adopts the character of its environment, which includes the soil. Soils that carry heavy metals, herbicides, pesticides, and waste can fill the plant with these undesirables. If the hemp is being used for fiber, its original use, there is no concern. But food-grade hemp to be used for nutrition, medicine, and beauty aids needs to be grown in pristine circumstances. In the United States, rules for agricultural health are stringent, and food-grade varieties of hemp are cultivated under the same guidelines as regular agricultural crops—ideally in certified-organic land. Always ask the manufacturer for documentation on the origin of the hemp they use.

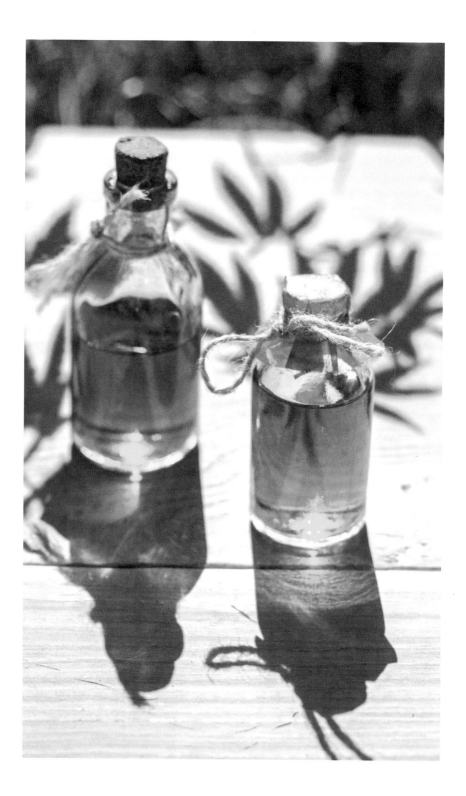

Know the Manufacturer

While hemp CBD products are gaining medicinal traction, they have yet to be produced by large, major pharmaceutical companies. In the meantime, small manufacturers are springing up to meet the growing demand. With many options on the market, it is important to investigate your options before you buy. Check a company's Better Business Bureau rating; then contact them directly to ask key questions, such as:

* What is their source of the CBD—both the kind of hemp plant used and its origin?

* How rigorously do they test for the contaminants mentioned above, as well as for bacteria and mold that may have been introduced during the manufacturing process?

* Do they do their own testing or send it to an independent lab? (Ideally the latter. Either way, be sure they or the lab are accredited and operate according to the ISO, or International Organization for Standardization.)

Finally, ask for a COA, or Certificate of Analysis. This will spell out the oil's origin and chemical content and confirm that it's contaminant-free. (See COA, page 52.) If a manufacturer cannot or will not answer these questions, it's time to move on.

Know Your CBD Language

It is important to understand the meaning of the following terms as they are commonly used when discussing CBD.

Aerial Plant Parts: The part of the plant above ground, including the stem, leaves, flowers, and branches.

Broad Spectrum: These hemp CBD products include all the phytocannabinoids and nutrients from the hemp plant, without any traces of THC.

COA: Certificate of Analysis, which is a government-rendered review of the contents of a CBD product.

Entourage Effect: Using products made with all the plant constituents has a more powerful healing effect than using products that isolate the CBD.

There are more than 100 other cannabinoids in hemp that support one another to increase their individual power. This yields a richer, more lasting healing effect.

Full Spectrum: This hemp CBD product contains many phytocannabinoids and other nutrients, including the maximum THC amount of 0.3 percent or less, per hemp's legal definition.

GMO: Genetically modified organisms, which include plants such as corn and soy whose natural makeup has been altered to resist insects and disease and may contain toxins.

ISO: International Organization for Standardization, which is responsible for setting batching standards and dosing levels.

Resin: Sticky, dew-like drops covering the marijuana plant, from which healing components are extracted to make medicine; hemp is not as rich in resin as is marijuana.

Know How to Read Labels

The label on your CBD product needs to be clear and complete. Here's a checklist to follow—and don't purchase a product until you're satisfied with each point. You may not be able to find every answer on the label, so be sure to talk with the manufacturer to receive the answers you want. Also speak with a health care professional to determine if the product's contents might cause an allergic reaction or work counter to a drug you are taking.

Batch number: This number displayed on the label ensures quality control. Using the batch number, you should be able to go on the manufacturer's website, locate the same number, and download the related COA (see definition on page 50).

CBD per dose: Look for the total amount of CBD in a bottle, as well as for the milligrams of CBD per recommended dose. If single dosage is not recommended, use the guidelines on page 54.

CBD-THC ratio: It is ideal to see the quantity and ratio of CBD to the THC trace amounts per dose. Many companies do not put "THC" on their labels because of fear of confusion by policing agencies. If that's the case, at least look for the amount of CBD per dose. If the label states only the full cannabinoid content (which includes CBD, THC, and other cannabinoids) per bottle, check with the manufacturer to clarify the CBD amount per dose.

COA: In addition to reading the label carefully, request a Certificate of Analysis (COA) from the manufacturer. Or, using the batch number, go to the manufacturer's website and pull up the certificate. The certificate, which comes after a review of the product by a third-party scientific laboratory, gives a full report on the product's origin, potency, terpene content, and purity, and lists contaminants such as pesticides and solvent residue.

Extraction method: Look first for CO_2 (either supercritical or subcritical) or food-grade ethanol extraction methods. Reject products whose methods used these toxic solvents: BHO, propane, or hexane.

List of active ingredients: Such a list can include herbal additives and pure flavorings like orange, mango, vanilla, or peppermint. Always reject products with preservatives, corn syrup, transfats, artificial coloring, GMOs, or thinning agents such as propylene glycol and ethylene glycol—often found in vape cartridges. If you are reading a long list of ingredients whose names you cannot pronounce, this is a sign that additives are replacing the quality of the CBD itself. Look elsewhere.

Manufacturing date: Be sure that the product bears a recent date and will not go bad before you've used it all. An unopened bottle generally will last 12–18 months and another 12 months once opened, as long as it is stored in a dark, cool cabinet or other place. If exposed to light or heat, or unused over time, it will grow rancid and need to be thrown out. Determine your use and buy accordingly. One recommendation is to buy a supply lasting 1–3 months at a time.

Origin and source of the hemp plant: Plants grown in states where cannabis is legal are the most tightly regulated. The plant should be grown specifically for CBD extraction, not the industrial hemp used for fiber or seeds, and should be organically, sustainably grown.

Plant parts used: The FDA requires a listing of the plant parts used to make the product, whether seeds, roots, or aerial portions, which include the stalk, leaves, and flowers. Not all manufacturers do this, so if it is not listed, either check with the manufacturer or move on.

Product manufacturer: Like the plant, products and their manufacturers from legal-cannabis states are held to high standards. To make sure a company is trustworthy, read up on it and call it if you have questions. If you have trouble reaching someone to answer your queries fully, go elsewhere.

Title: The label may call it "Hemp CBD Oil" or simply "CBD." Or, if there's a legal question about using the term "CBD" in a certain state, the title may be just "Hemp Oil." Always speak to the manufacturer if you have questions about the kind of product or its content.

Type of extract: The top two mainstream types are labeled as "full spectrum" and "broad spectrum" (for definitions, see pages 50–51). The lesser-known extract called "isolate" indicates that all plant compounds other than CBD have been removed.

Unfounded claims: Labeling that has a manufacturer's specific health claims are forbidden by the FDA. If the label declares that this product specifically heals arthritis or another condition, it should be a red flag.

KNOW HOW CBD MAY AFFECT YOU

Before you decide to use a CBD product, be aware that the treatment affects everyone in a different way. Your reaction to this or any new treatment will depend on your individual makeup, and that includes how your endocannabinoid receptors are concentrated in your individual body systems; so one body with arthritis might react to a small dose of CBD while another body with the same condition would need a larger dose. It also depends on the concentration and makeup of the product you buy. While CBD is not intoxicating, it may prompt a state of relaxation and calm that could, surprisingly, unnerve you. In this mental and physical state, you'd generally have no problem maintaining focus and continuing your daily routines—working, driving, caring for your family. If you're very sensitive, however, even the slightest THC content—0.3 percent for legal CBD—may prompt mental or emotional effects.

DOSAGE GUIDELINES

There is no single dosage guideline that covers every product and every person. The dosage that's right for you depends on the product, its concentration, your body, and the ailment you're trying to address. When you commit to using a hemp CBD supplement, you commit to working with a CBD-savvy health care professional to customize your optimal dosage. Caution is advised for those planning to take a higher-THC version of a CBD supplement than one with the legal 0.3 percent THC content. But caution spells success in the long run—and that's for everyone:

* Talk to your health care professional about your condition and why you'd like to start using hemp CBD to treat it. Be sure the doctor is CBD-aware. Deanna Gabriel Vierck notes: "In the herbal world, and particularly the cannabis herbal world, it is often recommended that the patient who wants to discuss CBD supplementation do their own research and bring copies of this info to the doctor's appointment. The reality is that most doctors are not well educated on herbal supplements and may have a bias against them. This is changing, and I think that patients helping to inform their doctors is a great part of this transition."

* Discuss other medications you may be taking and possible drug interactions. Be open about a history of drug or alcohol abuse, and determine together whether CBD is safe for your long-term use.

* Determine the delivery method that makes the most sense for you and your needs, whether a sublingual spray, a capsule, or any of the other products listed in this chapter.

* Titrate, titrate, titrate. That's the term for starting at a low dose and building up to the dose that works for you. This gives your body time to adjust and make optimal use of the CBD.

* Balance your needs with the basic information on the product label. If, for instance, the recommended dose for a CBD concentrate in a dropper bottle is 4–16 milligrams, twice a day, first be sure you know the amount delivered in a dropperful (see Dosing by Label, page 57). Next,

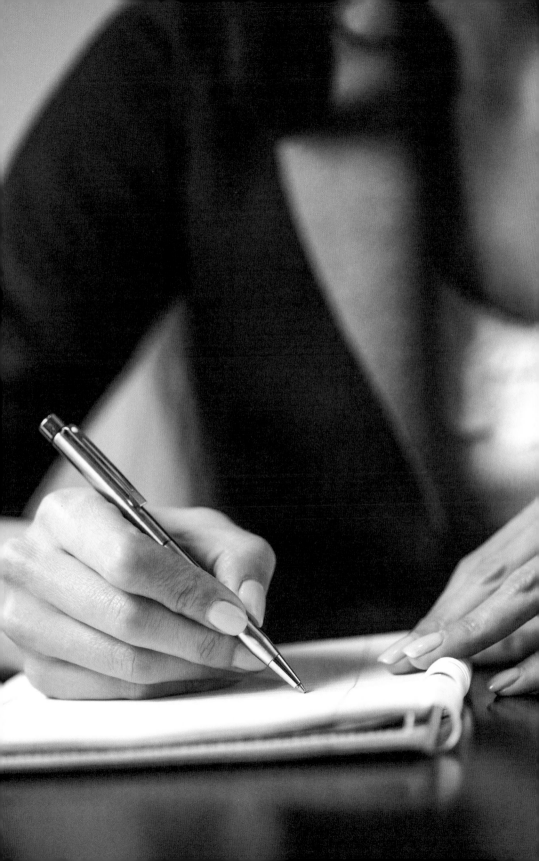

begin with 4 milligrams twice a day for four to five days. For the next four to five days, you might try 8 milligrams twice a day, building up, or titrating, to 16 milligrams twice a day. You may find that you need less than the maximum dosage stated on the label, or perhaps more.

* If you have reached the maximum recommended dosage, check in with your health care professional to discuss next steps. You may gradually move up the dosage ladder, but bear in mind that 50 milligrams twice a day—a total of 100 milligrams—or more is considered a high dosage.

* If at any time you feel a negative effect—perhaps extreme drowsiness or detoxing discomfort like nausea or headache—it is recommended that you return to a lower dose for a few days. Then cautiously return to the higher dose. Side effects are rare with CBD that contains 0.3 percent THC or less, but with highly absorbed products like nano-liposomal drops, you may experience nausea or headache detox symptoms; these often disappear as you drink extra water.

* While there are no known harmful side effects to hemp CBD products with 0.3 percent THC or less, it is still important to titrate slowly. Experts have found that less is sometimes more, and that the smaller dose can be just as effective as a larger dose—it will last longer, too. CBD from the marijuana plant, with higher levels of intoxicating THC, can have an effect that's called "biphasic." This means that the good feeling you get when first taking it can become a bad feeling when you take too much because it felt so good. Drinking alcohol is another biphasic example. Although hemp CBD is rarely biphasic, a slow, small start is always a good approach.

* Keep a journal that records your daily dosage; how your body is reacting—positively or negatively; what changes you are making in your routine; and how your attitude and energy are responding throughout the day.

* If CBD appears to be interacting negatively with your other medications, discontinue CBD use immediately.

In the end, effective dosing is as much about you as it's about the medicine. The consistent message is to go slowly and listen to your body.

Dosing by Label

Sometimes labels—even for excellent products—don't give you specific dosing information. Because many CBD supplements come in 1-ounce dropper bottles, here we offer the basic steps for determining dosage. This example considers that you want to begin with a low dosage of between 4 and 8 milligrams. It uses a bottle with a concentration of 250 milligrams of CBD per one ounce of product. Other one-ounce bottles will hold lower or higher concentrations of CBD. Adjust accordingly.

If the label reads: 250 mg CBD / 1 ounce

* There's a total of 250 milligrams of CBD in the entire one-ounce (30 ml) bottle.
* To determine the number of 4-milligram doses in the bottle: Divide 250 milligrams by 4 milligrams.
* There are about 60 (4-milligram) doses per bottle OR 30 (8-milligram) doses.

Now use the dropper to deliver the dose:

* In a one-ounce bottle, each dropperful holds $\frac{1}{30}$ ounce.
* Therefore, the entire bottle has 30 dropperfuls.
* If the bottle holds 250 milligrams of CBD, each dropperful holds about 8 milligrams of CBD.
* If taking 4 milligrams, your dose will be ½ dropperful. As you titrate up, 1 dropperful delivers 8 milligrams.

Dropper conversions:

* 1 dropperful = $\frac{1}{30}$ ounce = 1 ml = ¼ teaspoon = 30 drops

CBD AND SAFETY

As we've said many times, always talk with your physician before using CBD products; read labels; know your supplements or prescribed drugs and confirm with your doctor and a CBD expert whether or not you can safely use CBD at the same time; and establish a dosage that works for you.

While use of CBD was once cautioned against for children, pregnant and breastfeeding women, and pets, many products are now being considered for such uses. These often do not include additional flavorings or other ingredients; a purer product lowers the possibility of allergic or other negative reaction. Deanna Gabriel Vierck, among others, especially sees a bright future for CBD products for pets—both for the pet's sake and as a portal through which people might learn about CBD for their own use. Always consult your CBD-savvy health care provider (or your pets'!) before using CBD for any of these categories.

Tips on Where to Purchase CBD

Now that you've discovered the basics of hemp CBD products, it's time to take the plunge and actually bring them into your home. Once a CBD product is in your care, be sure to take care of it. If you work for it, it will work for you. These are a few common places that might carry CBD products in your area.

Dispensaries: If you live in one of the states where marijuana is legal, you may be able to buy a hemp CBD product in a dispensary. However, in some states, like Colorado, you can only buy hemp CBD in a health food store or boutique; the CBD products found in dispensaries are made from marijuana strains and will likely have enough THC—more than 0.3 percent— to cause some degree of intoxication. If you do go to a dispensary for CBD products, you'll have to bring an ID to show that you're at least 21 years of age in order to make a purchase. Ask all the same questions, ask for a tester, and be sure you're comfortable with the labeling and the manufacturer. Remember that unless the label indicates just 0.3 percent THC content or less, you can't carry these products across state lines.

Health Food Stores and Boutiques: Across the United States, health food stores and boutiques are beginning to stock sections with CBD supplements and other products made specifically from hemp. Before making a purchasing decision, ask to speak to the store buyer and to review the brands. Proprietors are excited about the growing interest in hemp CBD, and they're learning all they can, too. They'll likely share testers and literature you can take home. Before you buy, though, look into the manufacturer and COA, and follow the steps under Know How to Read Labels on page 51.

Online: In ways, this is your fastest bet. Although you won't have a face-to-face consultation or a tester, you'll be able to immediately look up the contents and the manufacturer's history, as well as the third-party lab and COA information. Calling the manufacturer can be more enlightening than speaking with a salesperson, too, unless that person is an expert.

Make Your Own Hemp CBD Oil? Not Right Now!

Some of you may be thinking: why spend a lot of money on a finished product when I can make my own CBD products, to my own specifications? First, growing hemp is illegal unless you're a certified research supplier; and those suppliers don't sell commercially. For those of you who are herb lovers, you've likely been out wildcrafting and have seen that a hemp-filled field has "healing" written all over it.

Even if you do get your hands on a hemp plant, a word of caution: Don't try it. Here's why: hemp that is grown for medicinal content needs to be grown in pristine surroundings. What you'll find in the field across the street, or even in a traditional hemp farm that grows hemp commercially for rope or canvas, is a plant likely filled with pesticides, herbicides, and other contaminants. For now, it's best to work with superbly formulated manufactured products.

Ready, Set, Go!

Starting a CBD regimen is a big commitment. Above, we've laid out the basics to help you understand CBD hemp products and how they can work for you. We've given you tips on where to buy and how to choose a product, read labels, and determine dosing.

In the following pages, we'll go deeper—into the individual ailments and conditions for which hemp CBD is increasingly becoming a go-to remedy. And we'll introduce you to some of the CBD-rich recipes we love.

We're glad you're along for the journey!

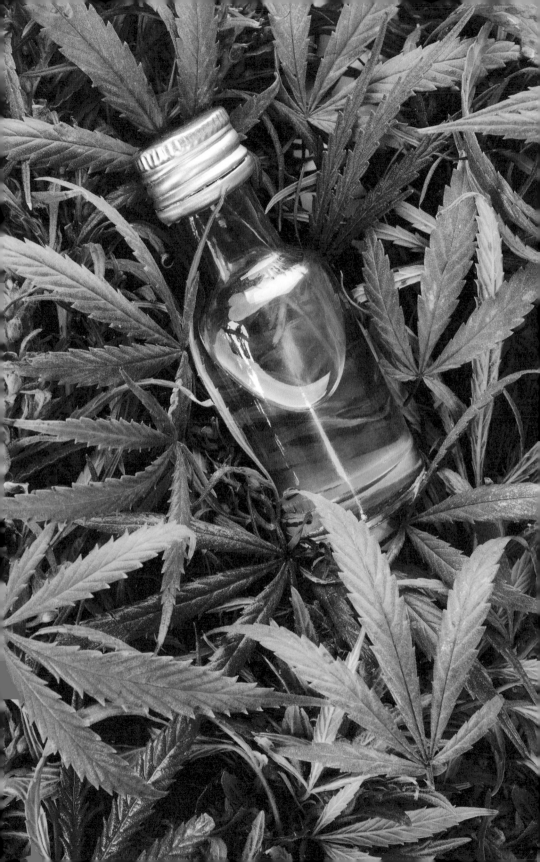

PART THREE

Ailments and Conditions

TREAT FIVE TO THRIVE . . .

Five key conditions are the main reasons you'll find CBD a healer for your body, mind, and soul. The first three, inflammation, stress, and insomnia, are the root causes of many of the other ailments we'll look at in this book. They are system-wide ailments that lower the body's natural ability to fight disease, detoxify, restore, and maintain balance. These three conditions immediately trigger two more: anxiety and depression. Together, this gang of five sets up your body as a revolving door, circulating illness in and out—and in. CBD's role as total-body remedy is to eliminate this three-plus-two equation from your life—and help you thrive.

For each of the five conditions below and for the 35 in the following section, we've given examples of how current research is finding CBD to work as a treatment. We also give a list of delivery systems for prompt uptake—either topical, ingested, or inhaled. While the fastest relief will likely come from using a trusted product directly from the package—according to the guidelines given by the manufacturer and your CBD-savvy health care professional—we also know that easing into CBD's use is important. That's why we've also given you recipes in Part Four that use CBD along with other delicious ingredients that support CBD's anti-inflammatory, antioxidant, and soothing powers.

NOTE: The potential delivery systems have been used with varying success and sometimes with THC combinations. Use of CBD depends on each individual's history, medication tolerance, size, and body weight. For many of the conditions, patients will already be taking other medications. Before using CBD, always consult a trusted, CBD-savvy health care expert to determine whether CBD is right for you and to determine the ideal delivery system and dosage—especially if you intend the use for a child or if you are pregnant.

THE THREE TRIGGERS

Inflammation

Experts will tell you that inflammation is the root of all evil. And science agrees. A certain amount of inflammation is key to healing: You cut yourself, and your immune system sends white blood cells rushing to the injured site; the area appears slightly red, puffy, and warm as the cells scramble to fight infection, sew up the ragged area with a scab, and gradually dissipate. Such healing of a contained incident—which could also be a sprained ankle, a stubbed toe, or a bout of bronchitis or acid reflux—is called acute inflammation. And it's what you want. Your immune system is acting in your best interest. You can help support it and speed up such healing by resting and protecting the area. If you don't allow acute inflammation to heal efficiently, the contained incident may be prolonged. Then it becomes chronic inflammation—and it can lead to bigger problems as your system works overtime to heal.

Chronic inflammation is triggered by free radicals. Simply put, these are atoms with unpaired electrons that the body generates when exposed to disease, environmental toxins, and poor diet. To become "whole," free radicals steal electrons from other molecules, starting a chain reaction of electron-nabbing that damages tissue. The body suffers oxidation—the same process that rusts a car or turns an apple slice brown. Oxidation also generates inflammation and vice versa. Chronic inflammation can lead to conditions that range from accelerated aging to digestive issues to cancer. In other cases, inflammation can be triggered when an imbalanced immune system attacks healthy tissue, as in rheumatoid arthritis and lupus. But most often, inflammation is the result of the next four aggravations—stress, insomnia, depression, and anxiety—and in turn causes them.

WHAT CBD CAN DO: CBD is found to help stimulate the endocannabinoid receptor CB2, which has protective anti-inflammatory effects. An NIH-supported study published in 2018 in the journal *Cannabis and Cannabinoid Research* reported that when CBD was used to relieve the inflammatory joint pain of arthritis, most patients reported it working "very well" or "moderately well" without the use of other supplemental drugs like over-the-counter ibuprofen or prescriptive steroids. By helping control inflammation, CBD may also help relieve inflammation's impact on cell oxidation, which promotes diabetes, Alzheimer's, high blood pressure, heart disease, and more.

DELIVERY SYSTEMS

* Ingested: capsules, concentrates, drops or sprays, edibles for long-term inner inflammatory conditions, nano/liposomal, sublingual tinctures.

* Topical: balms, lotions for muscle and joint concerns, oils, patches for skin, salves.

Stress

In the right doses, stress is a lifesaver and a gift. In a potentially dangerous situation, the nervous system, which keeps us at a level of regular operation (rest and digest), goes into hyperdrive (fight or flight), causing heart rate and blood pressure to rise and senses to sharpen. Suddenly your blood flows only to organs essential for quick response: brain, heart, and skeletal muscles. You think and act quickly to survive, and you are "on." But imagine what happens when you're "on" all the time. That's when merciful stress becomes a killer. Being in a demanding job or a rocky relationship can produce chronic stress overload that strains every organ in the body. It aggravates disorders that may exist, triggers new ones, and generally breaks down healthy operations, including tissue repair, digestive function, and detoxification pathways. You may take pride in your ability to manage a high-stress lifestyle, but it can also interrupt your healthy intentions of eating, sleeping well, and exercising regularly. The stress buildup not only can lead to anxiety and acute anxiety attacks, but over time it can take its toll on your health and long life as it catalyzes other ailments you'll see on the following pages.

WHAT CBD CAN DO: Chronic stress has been shown to alter and decrease endocannabinoid activity and tone—or its well-balanced operation. CBD, along with certain other beneficial hemp plant chemicals called terpenes, may help boost endocannabinoid function and effect its release of the soothing natural chemicals serotonin and dopamine through the 5-HT1A receptor. In her practice, says Deanna Gabriel Vierck observes, "I typically hear people say that while taking CBD they generally feel a greater sense of resilience during stress experiences at home and work, managing them with greater calm and clarity, and with fewer outbursts related to being frustrated and overwhelmed."

DELIVERY SYSTEMS

* Ingested: capsules, sublingual concentrates, drops or sprays, nano/ liposomal, or edibles for long-term stress reduction.

* Inhaled: vaporizing pen for immediate relaxation.

* Topical: salves, balms, lotions, oils to massage for relaxation.

Sleep Deprivation

Researchers have discovered that if you could package sleep into a capsule, you'd have a one-stop remedy that could help improve memory; boost problem-solving, learning, and memory; protect your immune system, heart, and libido; and control weight. Insomnia, the inability to sleep, affects millions of Americans—women more than men. Sleep—regulated by the endocannabinoid system—is how we regroup, remember, and heal: toxins are removed from the body, tissue is repaired, memories are stored, immunity is built, and so much more. In 2018, the American Sleep Association reported that as many as 70 million Americans suffer from insomnia and other sleep disorders, including snoring, sleep disruption, and sleep apnea. The result is that sufferers get less than the optimal

TESTIMONIAL

**Sarah McNaughton, mom, marketing professional
on stress, insomnia, and depression**

"When I first had my kids—now ages 6 and 11—I felt 'off' emotionally. I didn't know if it was hormonal or just becoming a mother," says Sarah McNaughton, a small business owner in Colorado. "First I had some depression with post partum; then I was easily agitated and angered by things. My littlest was in her tantrum stage, and I was very reactionary—I'd yell and fly off the handle. It would scare me. I was never physical, but I was having a really hard time controlling my emotions. Anger gave rise to guilt and shame and depression, like the world coming to an end. On top of that, I wasn't sleeping through the night. I'd wake up, and my mind was too active to get back to sleep. One day my brother suggested I try CBD. For the first few days I didn't feel anything; then after 5–6 days of taking drops 2–3 times a day, my mind started to quiet down. I became totally present inside—it had been so long since I'd felt that way. And I was sleeping through the night. One day while I was feeling this state of calm, my daughter started throwing a fit. Instead of screaming at her, I actually laughed! I knelt down on her level and calmly asked her, 'What do you need?' She just wanted a hug, a story, my attention. *Since taking CBD, I have an inner feeling of power and confidence. I know that whatever comes my way, I can handle it with a clear mind and calm body. I can figure out a solution.*"

seven to eight hours of sleep each night. This compromises quality of life and jeopardizes health. Over time, researchers have linked lack of sleep to increase in falls, car accidents, infections, depression, diabetes, high blood pressure, heart disease, concentration, and sex drive. Why can't we sleep? It could be light pollution from a clock radio or a cell phone, or overstimulation from exercise or from watching television too close to bedtime. It's also linked to health conditions such as stress, anxiety, depression, cough, menopausal night sweats, and frequent urination from enlarged prostate. Taking over-the-counter medications has its own side effects, including daytime fatigue, constipation, and liver damage. According to the National Sleep Foundation's 2018 poll, 90 percent of the people who prioritize sleep and sleep well reported feeling very effective at getting things done each day.

WHAT CBD CAN DO: While a 2014 animal study in the *Journal of Neuropharmacology* found that CBD can sometimes energize instead of promote sleep, its main benefits are promoting relaxation and sleep. As a sleep aid, CBD supports endocannabinoid receptors to reduce stress and anxiety, key to getting shut-eye. A 2016 animal study published in *PLoS ONE* journal showed that CBD's interaction with the endocannabinoid system promoted sleep stability and REM (rapid eye movement) sleep.

DELIVERY SYSTEMS

* Ingested: capsule, sublingual tincture, concentrate, spray or drop, nano/liposomal oil, isolates, edibles to help relieve other symptoms over time, in order to promote sleep. (Taken specifically for sleep, it can sometimes promote wakefulness.)

* Inhaled: vaporizing pen can relax before bedtime.

* Topical: salves, balms, lotions, oils to massage into temples to promote a restful state; most effective when combined with internal use.

THE TWO COMPLICATIONS

Anxiety

Anxiety happens, and as with stress, our system steps in to help us manage anxious times, and healthful living helps promote calm and balance. But anxiety is elusive. With stress, once you've identified its cause, you can often take steps to adjust your lifestyle; even if it takes a while, you have some sense of control. Symptoms of anxiety, however, may surprise you suddenly in the form of a panic attack with chest pain, sweating, and heart palpitations; an obsessive-compulsive activity; or a phobia, perhaps of a crowded room or a spider. Once triggered, these attacks can return again and again, becoming chronic and almost impossible to control. They may limit your ability to socialize, interact at work, and even walk down a crowded city sidewalk. Anxiety conditions, such as post-traumatic stress (PTS) and social anxiety disorder (SAD), are among those anxieties that attack 18 percent of adults across the nation in any given year, says the National Institute of Mental Health (NIMH). You'll learn more about these specific anxiety disorders
and others on the following pages.

WHAT CBD CAN DO: As with stress, CBD also works to help the 5-HT1A receptor release calming serotonin and dopamine. Two terpenes in the hemp plant support this action: Limonene, also prevalent in citrus and responsible for its scent, is known to improve mood; and linalool, a component of lavender, is hailed as a stress reliever and anxiety calmer. Results of a Dutch study published in 2017 in the *Cannabis and Cannabidiol Research* journal indicated that human subjects had lower levels of anxiety and confusion and increased alertness, tranquility, and confidence after using CBD.

DELIVERY SYSTEMS

* Ingested: capsule, sublingual tincture, concentrate, spray or drop, nano/liposomal oil, isolates, or edibles to help elevate mood.
* Inhaled: vaporizing pen for immediate anxiety attack relief.

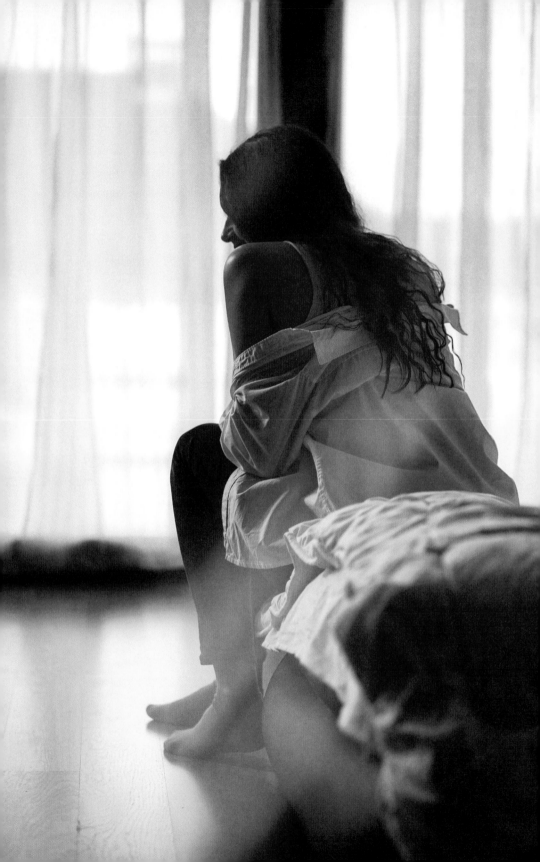

Depression

Everyone experiences sadness. It's a normal part of life, and your sadness needs to be indulged as you work toward getting back on your feet. It may take weeks or sometimes months depending on the situation, but during this time you will also find positive aspects of life and see the light ahead. In some cases, however, profound sadness will continue indefinitely. You may find it hard to enjoy people, activities, and events. You may feel worthless, guilty, tired, or irritable, with unexplained outbursts of anger or tears. You may be unable to sleep, eat, or focus. Thoughts of suicide may visit. If you're persistently experiencing such symptoms, listen closely: Seek professional help. Your quality of life—and perhaps life itself—are in jeopardy, because you're opening the door to heart disease, stroke, and other chronic conditions triggered by this one. Above all, know that you are not alone. In 2017, the World Health Organization reported that more than 300 million people around the world suffer from depression. Health care professionals are there, working overtime to guide you.

WHAT CBD CAN DO: As with stress and anxiety, depression may be related to poor endocannabinoid tone and function. Studies show that, like commercial antidepressants, CBD may enhance the receptors that release soothing dopamine and serotonin. Results from animal tests published in *Current Pharmaceutical Design* in 2014 noted that CBD taken consistently could mimic successful antidepressants by enhancing CB1 receptors. A 2016 study with mice published in *Neuropharmacology* noted that CBD "exerts fast and antidepressant effects" and "significantly enhanced levels of serotonin," likely by interacting with 5-HT1A receptors. The other highly important point is that CBD exerts these positive effects *without* the negative side effects of many prescription drugs, which can include dry mouth, constipation, and nausea.

DELIVERY SYSTEMS

* Ingested: capsule, sublingual tincture, concentrate, spray or drop, nano/liposomal oil, edibles to help elevate mood and possibly sleep (for some it causes wakefulness); hemp seed oil drops rich in omega-3s can enhance benefits.

* Inhaled: vaporizing pen for mild mood change and sleep.

...AND 35 MORE TO SCORE

Below you'll find 35 conditions related to the five umbrella conditions on the previous pages. You'll find that CBD is either being actively used or studied to address each one—and that CBD may have a role in your future or a loved one's. More important, you'll discover that CBD is just part of the equation for maintaining a lifestyle that supports health and fends off disease. Remember the integrative approach to total health we discussed on pages 21–24. Then read on.

Addiction: Smoking, Alcohol, Drugs

Addiction to smoking, alcohol, and drugs, especially opiates including morphine and fentanyl, are at an epidemic level in the United States today. As any one of these toxins interacts with receptors in the endocannabinoid system, it changes mood and produces a high, a welcome feeling of reward, for a short amount of time. Once that dissipates, the need for reward comes back more insistently—with a vengeance. According to the Centers for Disease Control, there are some 38 million smokers across the nation and smoking is a leading cause of heart disease, lung cancer, and a multitude of other ailments. In 2015, opioid overdose caused 33,000 deaths in the United States, according to the National Institutes of Health, and in 2018 approximately 115 people died each day. Opioid consumption often begins as a prescriptive medicine for persistent pain and then becomes a dependency that gradually leads to death, often because the lungs shut down. And alcoholism continues to thrive in this fast-paced environment where exhausted workers, parents, and students choose relaxation through drink instead of sleep and exercise. While a glass of wine may be a welcome soother at the end of a hard day, a bottle of wine is not. Like other addictive substances, it is biphasic: a little may be good, but the "good" leads us to consume more to feel "better." Unfortunately, the more you consume, the worse you feel and the more harm it does to your body. Beyond leading you to say and do things you wish you hadn't, alcohol overconsumption breaks down tissues and organs, leading to disease, from throat cancer to liver cirrhosis.

WHAT CBD CAN DO: Above all, CBD helps you avoid addiction in the first place, by soothing the five umbrella conditions that often spark it— inflammation, stress, insomnia, anxiety, and depression. However, research shows that once addiction sets in, CBD has great potential value for addressing all forms of addictive behavior. The interesting thing is that CBD can also help reduce the dependency on its sister cannabinoid, intoxicating THC. This is how scientists think it works: The endocannabinoid receptors play a big role in how we respond to reward. The immediate reward a person feels upon taking a pill, a drink, or a smoke helps lead them down an addictive path. Studies increasingly show that CBD may play a role in blocking the receptors that produce that feeling of reward. And it likely helps deliver serotonin to relieve the anxiety and insomnia that accompany withdrawal. Fortunately, while the endocannabinoid system is central to the addicting sensation of reward, it also helps reset brain circuitry and promote healing. CBD is a key player in both these paths.

DELIVERY SYSTEMS

* Ingested: capsule, sublingual tincture, concentrate, spray or drop, nano/liposomal oil, edible for withdrawal symptoms of nausea, vomiting, anxiety, headache, appetite loss, and perceived pain.

* Inhaled: vaporizing pen for anxiety, especially early in withdrawal process.

Antiaging

While growing older brings knowledge and wisdom, no one looks forward to the bodily aging that comes with it. Still, it can't be stopped, and the best way to face it is to keep your body as toned as you can, from your brain to the minutest muscle. That includes endocannabinoid tone, or balance (see page 19). Aging seems to be the result of free radicals that trigger oxidation throughout our bodies. Oxidation damages cells and tissue, causing inflammation and chronic illness that lead to aging. It affects our brains as dementia, skin as wrinkles, joints as arthritis, and blood vessels as vascular and heart disease. Frontline therapy is refreshingly natural: Fruits and vegetables are packed with antioxidants, which strengthen cells, support new cell growth, and counter tissue-damaging free radicals; they also have cell-protective vitamins A, C, D, and more. Fish and nuts deliver omega-3 fatty acids, which support brain health; and water keeps every part of our body hydrated and flushes our system of toxins. Exercise, too, is a proven antiaging force. Researchers have found that exercise not only improves circulation and builds strong heart and lung capacity, but it even builds brain cells. Avoiding smoking, too much sun, and stress in your life contribute to this natural fountain of youth. Such a conscientious lifestyle carries its own "entourage effect"—and CBD and other hemp constituents contributes to it as well.

WHAT CBD CAN DO: For centuries, hemp seed oil, different from hemp CBD oil, has been used to nourish skin, our largest organ. Its omega-6 and omega-3 fatty acids help make skin moist and supple; its antioxidant vitamin E helps reduce age lines and encourages new skin and hair cells to grow. More recently its cousin, CBD has become a go-to product for antioxidant and anti-inflammatory properties that not only enhance skin tone as a topical application but also support endocannabinoid tone and body-wide cell protection when taken internally. Its antiaging potential is great, with studies that show its success in the fight against smoking addiction (which turns us old overnight), diabetes, age-related memory loss, bone loss, eye disease, arthritis, and neurological movement disorders like Parkinson's.

DELIVERY SYSTEMS

* Ingested: capsule, sublingual tincture, concentrate, spray or drop, nano/liposomal oil, or edible to promote resilience from within.
* Topical: salves, balms, lotions, oils for skin protection and flourishing.

Antibiotic-Resistant Bacterial Infection

Bacterial infections come in many forms: An uncovered cut may ulcerate. Strep throat, which is common in children, may strike during flu season. Or a staph infection like impetigo, cellulitis, or a boil, all of which cause redness, swelling, and oozing, can easily be passed from person to person through sports equipment, gym towels, and even hotel sheets. (Such bacteria are so tough they can resist cleaning!) Bacterial poisoning from contaminated food or water is all too frequent. When you're healthy and you develop a bacterial infection, you may think that good care and possibly an antibiotic will quickly clear it up. In many cases, it does. In others, especially if your immune system is not up to snuff, the bacteria can spread throughout your body and turn deadly. A well-known example is the bacterial strain called Methicillin-resistant *Staphylococcus aureus* (MRSA), which has shown up in hospitals around the world, infecting both patients and healthy people around them. This superbug has a Hulk-like exterior that makes once-healing drugs bounce off it like Ping-Pong balls. In a race to arrest this villain and others, scientists and doctors have been testing and using CBD and other cannabinoids. The results are promising.

WHAT CBD CAN DO: Experts are finding that the antiseptic properties in CBD and other cannabinoids can help fight vicious bacterial infections resistant to antibiotics. A study by Italian scientist Giovanni Appendino published in the *Journal of Natural Products* in 2008 noted that several cannabinoids "showed potent antibacterial properties" and that healing from MRSA increased when topical CBD products were applied to ulcers and wounds. CBD has also been used orally to fight internal infection. Researchers are still working to identify how, exactly, it targets and shuts down bacterial activity, but they report positive findings in NIH-supported studies from 2016 and 2017. In addition, researchers have found that the terpene pinene, which accompanies CBD in the hemp plant, not only has antibacterial properties but also permeates the skin quickly, reaching the bloodstream for extra-fast delivery.

DELIVERY SYSTEMS

* Ingested: capsule, sublingual tincture, concentrate, spray or drop, nano/liposomal oil, edible to fight internal infection.
* Topical: salves, balms, lotions, oils for external infection.

Arthritis

Are your joints stiff and swollen? Are you experiencing mild or severe pain in your fingers, knees, or back? You may be among the 54 million adults across the United States who, the Arthritis Foundation tells us, have been diagnosed with arthritis—with a projected 78 million by 2040. Sadly, arthritis also affects some 300,000 American children. Generally speaking, arthritis causes the joints to become inflamed and lose function. Symptoms include joint stiffness and swelling, low-grade aches, and chronic pain. There are more than a hundred kinds of arthritis—including those triggered by Lyme disease and lupus—but the two most common are osteoarthritis and rheumatoid arthritis. Osteoarthritis develops from natural overuse of joints through time and can be exacerbated by weight and injury. Rheumatoid arthritis is an autoimmune disorder; the body's immune system attacks membranes in the joints, inflaming them until they're damaged, making each movement agony. There's no cure for these painful conditions. Acetaminophen, which helps lower fever, is a long-time arthritis pain reliever, but overuse can hurt the liver or kidney; steroids offer efficient relief, but side effects can range from infection to decrease in bone density. While it's painful to move, movement in fact is key: both physical therapy and exercise in general can help relieve symptoms.

WHAT CBD CAN DO: In a 2006 study published in the journal *Rheumatology*, the cannabis-based medicine Sativex® (also found helpful for multiple sclerosis, page 107) was reported to lessen joint pain in arthritis sufferers. However, with its 1:1 ratio of THC to CBD, Sativex has not been approved for use in the United States. Since then, deeper research into CBD has found that it helps boost the number of endocannabinoids created naturally in the body's ECS; these in turn interact with CB1 and CB2 receptors in the nervous and immune system to control inflammation and immune response. A 2010 study published in *Future Medical Chemistry* reported that both THC and CBD may help suppress cytokines, inflammatory proteins released by the immune system. For an entourage effect, scientists report that the terpene BCP, or beta-carophyllene, found in hemp as well as in black pepper and rosemary, likely supports CBD's anti-inflammatory effects. Finally, CBD has been found to promote the regeneration of bone tissue in bones damaged by arthritis. (See Bone Health and Osteoporosis, page 81.)

* Ingested: capsule, sublingual tincture, concentrate, spray or drop, nano/liposomal oil, or edible to help address long-term pain, inflammation, and tissue and bone damage.

* Inhaled: vaporizing pen for acute pain.

* Topical: salves, balms, lotions, oils, transdermal patches help address pain.

Asthma

America's most chronic childhood disease—and the top reason for missed school days—is the inflammatory condition called asthma. Poor diet, obesity, and indoor air filled with dust, mold, and pet dander can be underlying causes. Or outdoor pollutants and allergens can trigger wheezing, chest tightening, and shortness of breath as air passages swell and fill with excessive mucus. A cough that's worse at night or in early morning can leave parents constantly on the alert. While a child may grow better as the lungs grow bigger, often it's a matter of learning to manage symptoms throughout a lifetime. According to the Asthma and Allergy Foundation of America, more than 26 million Americans of all ages suffer from asthma. Women suffer more than men, and prevalence is greatest in African American and Puerto Rican communities. Most often asthma's origin is a combination of genetic and environmental factors. So while it may be encoded in your system, you can learn to navigate through challenging times. Knowing the catalysts, aside from allergies, is key: an attack may be set off by a respiratory infection; a change in temperature or humidity; strenuous exercise; or sudden anger, fear, or shock. A bronchodilator is the frontline tool for opening the airways and arresting an attack. For chronic and severe conditions, a health care professional will likely prescribe a medicine to inhale or take orally. Following the doctor's regimen precisely can be a matter of life or death. Building a strong body and immune system is key: experts may recommend a vegan or vegetarian diet void of allergy-inducing milk and eggs, massage therapy, acupuncture, or yoga and other moderate exercise to strengthen the lungs.

WHAT CBD CAN DO: Through animal test results published in medical journals in 2008 and 2012, scientists identified that CB1 and CB2 receptors in bronchial tissue—the main passageway to the lungs—keep the lungs healthy. In case of irritation, the receptors were shown to help dilate, or open, airways. CB2 receptors were especially shown to play a part in lowering inflammation. While THC has been the most studied cannabinoid in boosting the work of these receptors, more recent studies published in 2015 show that CBD supports their anti-inflammatory effort, helps reduce mucus secretion that blocks airways, and helps relieve the anxiety that accompanies an attack. (See Anxiety, page 67.)

NOTE: The cannabis plant can prompt allergies in some people, and a possible asthma attack. Approach usage carefully and, as always, talk to your CBD-savvy medical professional, especially if using a separate medication for asthma.

DELIVERY SYSTEMS

* Ingested: capsule, sublingual tincture, concentrate, spray or drop, nano/liposomal oil, or edible to ease long-term inflammation and help dilate airways for improved airflow. It's best to avoid alcohol-based tinctures in children.

* Inhaled: vaporizing pen for potential relief of immediate symptoms—but starting with extremely small doses and watching for allergic reaction.

Attention-Deficit/Hyperactivity Disorders: (ADHD, also called ADD, Attention Deficit Disorder)

In this day and age it often seems impossible to concentrate: you're being friended, or a new social media post is demanding your attention. Most people gradually learn to balance the continuous pinging, to take what they need and ignore what they don't. But for those with attention-deficit/hyperactivity disorder (ADHD), that's another story. Generally diagnosed in childhood, ADHD is characterized by a person's inability to pay attention and to sit still. It can be mild or severe. A mild form of hyperactivity can simply mean daydreaming, easy distraction, and forgetfulness. If severe, it may include impulsive and sometimes uncontrollable fidgeting or motion, excessive talking, even screaming. Or there's a combination of the two. While ADHD is widely diagnosed in school-aged children, some 2–5 percent of adults also have it. There is no definitive cause, but experts have linked the development of ADHD to genetics, premature birth, an environment filled with lead or other toxins, or a diet rich in sugars and transfats at the expense of one rich in brain-powering omega-3 fatty acids. Whatever the root, it appears that the brain is overwhelmed by incoming information. Instead of efficiently sifting through and addressing incoming signals, it suffers information overload. In addition, scientists have found that the brain is not naturally generating the calming drug dopamine. Traditional drugs like Ritalin® and Adderall® help the brain release dopamine, but they may also cause side effects like insomnia, stomachache, mood swings, and deeper psychiatric conditions.

WHAT CBD CAN DO: Pioneer in cannabis research and a longtime advocate of substance abuse programs Dr. David Bearman has led the way in studying the interaction of cannabinoids with the endocannabinoid system—and their effect on ADHD. His results have shown that cannabinoids help support the production of soothing dopamine, which helps the brain regulate information input and aids in calming and focus. While his work is marijuana-centric, more recent studies look to the non-psychoactive effects of CBD as well. A 2017 *Neuro Image: Clinical* article holds that cannabinoids have neuroprotective benefits, key to ADHD control.

DELIVERY SYSTEMS

* Ingested: capsule, sublingual tincture, concentrate, spray or drop, nano/liposomal oil, edible for potential to promote mind clarity and focus.

* Inhaled: vaporizing pen for calming and clarity.

Autism

This umbrella classification covers neurobehavioral conditions that may range from being gifted but having difficulties in socializing—apparent in a kind called Asperger's syndrome—to severe disorders that may include lack of speech and communication, repetitive behavior, and violent outbursts. According to the Centers for Disease Control, 1 in 59 children in the United States is diagnosed with autism. There is no cure. Sometimes symptoms

Deanna Gabriel Vierck, CCH CN, clinical herbalist and clinical nutritionist

The Healing Mindset

Taking CBD can create profound changes in physical health for some. While this may *sound* welcome and wonderful, it requires a rewiring of our inner world and a need to focus on healing our hearts and human spirits so we can maintain this new way of being. I have seen people experience results from CBD supplementation that seem miraculous, only to find that several months later they had stopped the CBD and were once again struggling. Why? Sometimes these supplements can be so powerful on a physical and emotional level that people aren't ready for the change—they feel more comfortable reverting to the life they know. As your physical body changes, you need to work hard to change your mental vision of yourself, too. If you don't, you'll hit a blockage and either slide back into the problem or create a new one. I believe true healing requires a willingness to adjust how you live your life and how you think of yourself. Are you *truly* willing to let go of your previous identity and actively create a new, healthier one? *Integrating therapeutic remedies like plants, healthy diet, exercise, spiritual work, and support groups into your lifestyle can help you achieve and maintain a higher level of vitality as you use CBD and could offer profound support as you allow the process of true, complete healing to unfold.*

are benign: failing to better fit in at a social function, missing conversational cues, or lacking empathy. Others are impossible to deal with: hyperactivity, tantrums, and self-harm, requiring some patients to be institutionalized. Causes of autism may be both genetic and environmental. Research published in a 2015 issue of the *International Journal of Epidemiology* suggests that a pregnant mother's use of alcohol and tobacco, her diet's lacking key nutrients like folate and fatty acids, and even her exposure to air pollution may all contribute to altered neurodevelopment. While behavioral therapy is often recommended as the core treatment, some pharmaceuticals used in conjunction with therapy have been found to alleviate irritability, reduce anxiety, or arrest seizures. The Autism Research Institute shares more than 40 years' worth of parent rankings of medicines, therapies, and diets they've found effective. Work continues on the potential for cannabis-centered relief.

WHAT CBD CAN DO: An early advocate of using cannabis in the form of THC was Dr. Bernard Rimland, founder of the Autism Research Institute, a psychologist with an autistic son. In the 1960s he pioneered autism treatments that included cannabis. Today, the institute records show examples of cannabis use related to reduction in anxiety, panic, aggression, and harmful behavior. Rimland's early work opened the door to understanding how the endocannabinoid system affects autism. Research in a 2015 *Neurotherapeutics* journal suggests that ECS receptors play a vital role in brain development, reward response, circadian rhythm, and anxiety—all disrupted or imbalanced in autism. THC's—also CBD's—interaction with these receptors may bring positive results—and hope. A 2017 *Journal of Pediatric Pharmacology and Therapeutics* issue notes that CBD's ability to calm epilepsy may make it a prime candidate for treating similar symptoms in autism. And an ongoing child-based study under Israeli neurologist Adi Aran gives CBD a big thumbs up: as of 2018, it shows "the feasibility of CBD-based medical cannabis as a promising treatment."

DELIVERY SYSTEMS

* Ingested: capsule, sublingual tincture, concentrate, spray or drop, nano/liposomal oil, or edible for long-term symptoms. It's best to avoid alcohol-based tinctures in children.

* Inhaled: vaporizing pen for immediate symptoms like anxiety or violent outburst, but for adults only.

Bladder Health and Incontinence

The uncomfortable result of an overactive bladder often comes calling as we age. Overactive bladder is a condition in which the bladder muscles involuntarily contract. Without warning, you may find yourself in an uncomfortable and embarrassing situation. Overactive bladder can also be the result of infection, a swollen prostate, a tumor, or a stone. Multiple sclerosis and Parkinson's—or any other neurological condition—can also trigger it. Finally, too much liquid intake, usually coffee or alcohol, may be the culprit. Noninvasive treatment begins with absorbent pads; Kegel exercises, which strengthen the pelvic floor muscle; scheduled bathroom trips; and maintaining healthy weight. Talk to your health care professional about the several medications on the market, and beware of their side effects.

Keeping your bladder infection-free is also key to healthy bladder activity. If you're a woman, you've probably experienced a bladder, or urinary tract, infection. This uncomfortable scenario can come from *E. coli* wiped forward after a bowel movement; from waiting too long to urinate or not completely voiding; and even from sexual intercourse, especially if you've failed to urinate immediately afterward. Women suffer most often from this: if infection enters the urethra, the short tube that sends urine from the kidneys to the genital opening, it quickly spreads to the bladder; if not treated, it can move upward to the kidneys. So act fast: extreme urgency, burning, fever, and pelvic ache require a doctor's visit and usually an antibiotic.

In middle-aged women, interstitial cystitis, or painful bladder syndrome, may feel like a urinary tract infection, with burning and a frequency of urinating up to 60 times a day. Doctors don't know what causes it, but they do know it's not bacterial and that antibiotics don't work. Some doctors have found that filling the bladder with a medicinal solution helps "wash" it out to relieve symptoms. There is no cure, but diet and exercise may help limit inflammation. On the next page, see what CBD and other cannabis studies are showing.

WHAT CBD CAN DO: Good news begins with the endocannabinoid system, where receptors in the nervous system and bladder keep muscles operating smoothly and urgency in check. A series of trials over a decade show that CBD has the potential to interact with these receptors to relax bladder muscles, lowering urgency and frequency. It may also relieve painful bladder syndrome. In a 2004 study, MS patients used a combination of CBD and THC to greatly improve comfort and sleep while decreasing urination—with few side effects; and a 2015 animal study focusing on CBD supported these findings. A 2014 *Journal of Urology* article sees the ECS as a target for lowering the inflammation of painful bladder syndrome—meaning the door is open to CBD healing.

DELIVERY SYSTEMS

* Ingested: capsule, sublingual tincture, concentrate, spray or drop, nano/liposomal oil, or edible for long-term symptoms including pain, inflammation, and bladder muscle contractions.

Bone Health and Osteoporosis

Bones are a beautiful thing: they are organs alive with tissue, blood, and minerals. We are born with rubbery, flexible bones. Through childhood and into our mid-30s, the bones harden as we generate new bone tissue, increasing density. After that, we begin to lose bone tissue more quickly than it can build up—and the bones need extra care through diet and exercise to remain strong. If they don't get it, they'll morph from hard to brittle through bone loss. This is more noticeable in women than in men. First, men simply begin life with greater bone density, so the loss appears more gradual, and second, a woman's rate of bone loss increases after menopause. Still, both males and females—in fact some 44 million people across the nation—suffer from osteoporosis. In this disease, the bones (os) become riddled with holes (porous). This is a silent disease, so you may not notice symptoms until you suddenly fracture your foot for no apparent reason. As you age, inform your doctor if you have a family history of osteoporosis or if you take medications that might trigger bone loss. Maintain a healthy weight: while being overweight can keep you from moving and building bone, being underweight means your body may be pulling vital minerals from your bones to maintain stability. Whatever the case, don't despair! At all ages, bone can renew and strengthen with a calcium- and vitamin D-rich diet and exercise that causes impact: walking, running, jumping, and lifting weights. If you're healthy, you'll prevent problems later. If you've discovered bone loss, get started now. And see below how CBD may help.

WHAT CBD CAN DO: In the early 2000s, researchers began to see how the endocannabinoid system plays a major role in regulating bone health. They identified CB2 receptors as supporting the production of minerals that build bone and slow down the work of resorption cells that instigates bone loss. A University of Tel Aviv animal study published in a 2015 *Journal of Bone and Mineral Research* (JBMR) showed that CBD helped increase collagen production to heal fractured bone and make it stronger. In 2016, researchers published findings indicating that the terpene BCP, useful in arthritis (see page 73), can stimulate mineral production of bone marrow and suppress bone loss in animals. The door is open for studies to determine how BCP may help prevent and treat osteoporosis in humans.

DELIVERY SYSTEMS

* Ingested: capsule, sublingual tincture, concentrate, spray or drop, nano/liposomal oil, or edible for long-term bone-building and protection.

Cancer and Chemotherapy

To get a handle on cancer, think about your cells. Every cell in the body has a lifespan: It generates, divides, becomes worn out, and dies as new cells take its place. Sometimes factors inside or outside the body prompt them to divide way too fast and grow out of control, crowding out normal cells and forming tumors. These in turn metastasize, or spread throughout the body. Cancer is America's number two killer—after heart disease. While you may know the common ones, like breast, prostate, lung, colon, and skin, the list includes more than 100—brain, bronchial, thyroid, and liver, to name a few. Few forms are hereditary; most are prompted by three main—and preventable—environmental factors: smoking; pollutants like radiation and factory toxins; and poor diet and obesity.

Katie Ortlip, RN, LCSW,
hospice expert for SHARECARE network, Dr. Ahmet Oz's
online health and wellness platform, and coauthor of
Living with Dying: A Complete Guide for Caregivers

CANCER

"Years ago when I started working in hospice, people were using marijuana with helpful medical results, but no one talked about it," says hospice social worker Katie Ortlip. "Now that medical marijuana and low-THC CBD are becoming mainstream, our hospice nurses are happy that it's more available, and many have CBD on their medications list. It's not unusual for patients to ask for it. Oil is the most popular of the products among the cookies, caramels, lotions, gels, and creams. Not long ago I had a patient more than 100 years old with advanced dementia, who was suffering from bedsores and moaning deep into the night—perhaps from pain or anxiety or both. Her daughter did not want to give her morphine, the usual prescription, so she began giving her mother a few drops of CBD oil at night. Soon we noticed that her mom was more relaxed, slept better, and didn't cry out. The daughter administered CBD until her mom passed away peacefully. Another patient had aggressive pancreatic cancer, the kind that leaves patients bedridden with only a month or so of life. But she remained very active for 7 months: she went camping several times with her husband and daughter and lived a high quality of life without the usual symptoms of pain and nausea. *She and her husband swore by CBD and said that it not only contributed to that high quality, but likely prolonged her life."*

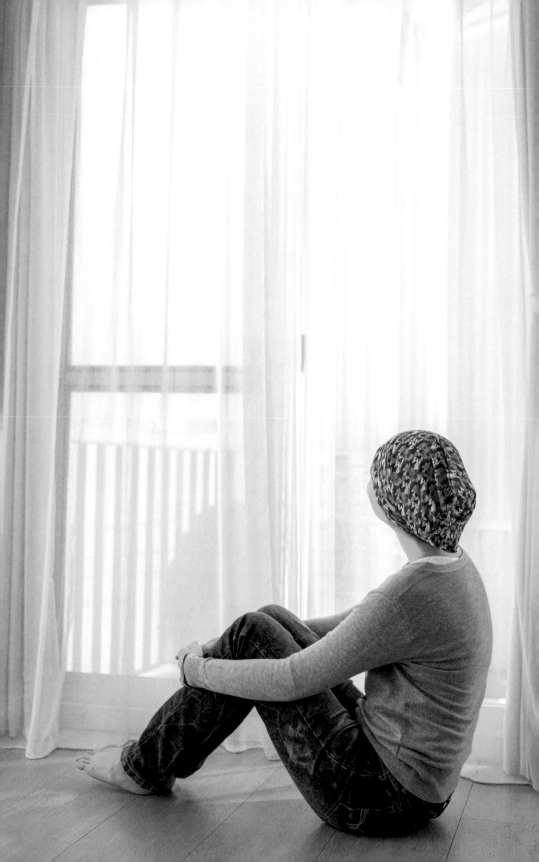

Alcoholism and lack of sleep contribute as well. In 2018, more than 1.5 million cases will have been diagnosed, says the National Institutes of Health. But their statistics also bring hope: some 16 million survivors thrive today, and their numbers are on the rise. While cancer survivors can tell you that cancer is never fully "cured," multiple treatments are available to put it in remission, depending on the type of cancer: surgery to remove a contained tumor, radiation to shrink it, hormone therapy to slow or stop growth, and chemotherapy, in which a chemical mixture in liquid, injection, pill, or topical form targets tumors and body-wide cancer cells. Radiation and chemotherapy come with side effects—fatigue, nausea and vomiting. In the future these side effects, along with the cancer itself, may be reduced because of CBD.

WHAT CBD CAN DO: For cancer patients, CBD can be an administering angel, improving quality of life by inducing sleep, calming anxiety, addressing nerve and other body pain, and stimulating appetite. Among its most welcome—and documented—roles is quelling the nausea and vomiting that accompanies chemotherapy. But can it *cure* cancer? There is no definitive evidence, and anyone shilling "the cure" deserves scrutiny. But scientists are working overtime to discern how CBD and other cannabinoids affect cancer. And research is plentiful: Among a score of major studies, a 2018 report in *Surgical Neurology International* holds that phytocannabinoids—mainly CBD and THC—show promise in killing cancer cells, inhibiting tumor growth, and halting metastasis, or spreading of cells—in glioma, lymphoma, prostate, breast, pancreatic, and colon cancers, among others. Research shows that CBD and THC work best in supporting roles—always continue your prescribed treatment—and when used together. While THC efficiently activates endocannabinoid receptors to catalyze the fight, CBD steps in as an effective reinforcement. In addition, terpenes in cannabis appear to join the tumor fight. Studies with limonene show its protective effects against tumor formation in the breast, pancreas, and other areas, and myrcene appears to slow abnormal cell growth.

DELIVERY SYSTEMS:

* Ingested: capsule, sublingual tincture, concentrate, spray or drop, nano/liposomal oil, or edible for pain and symptoms according to each kind of cancer, as well as for nausea and vomiting from chemotherapy.

* Inhaled: vaporizing pen for immediate pain and nausea relief.
* Topical: salves, balms, lotions, oils for bruising and skin changes that come with some cancer treatments.

Diabetes

If you're one of the more than 30 million people who suffer from diabetes, you're constantly aware of what you eat, how you exercise, and especially how you watch your insulin levels. Insulin is the operative word here. It's what diabetes is all about. Insulin is a hormone produced by the pancreas, and its main function is to transfer glucose, or sugar, from the bloodstream into fat, muscle, and liver cells. Without its moderating effects, levels of blood glucose can skyrocket, damaging tissue and starving cells. In type 1 diabetes, which usually is diagnosed in childhood, the pancreas fails to make adequate insulin. This may be due to a genetic condition in which antibodies attack the cells that produce insulin. In type 2 diabetes, the pancreas produces the right amounts of insulin, but the fat, muscle, and liver cells don't respond to it; they are resistant. This version has to do with lifestyle, so take a good look at yours. Are you overweight or obese? Sleep-starved? A walking stress machine? A couch potato? Each contributes to making insulin-resistant cells. If you're any one of these or if you have a family history of diabetes, reassess your lifestyle. Diabetes is not self-contained; sustained high blood sugar can age tissue, damage blood vessels and nerves, promote heart disease and stroke, and lead to retinopathy, the number one most preventable cause of blindness in adults, according to the National Institutes of Health.

WHAT CBD CAN DO: CBD appears to be useful for both type 1 and type 2 diabetes. In the case of type 1, it may interact with ECS receptors to help lower inflammation in the pancreas and effect insulin production. In type 2 diabetes, findings published in a 2012 *American Journal of Pathology* concluded that, rather than acting through receptors, CBD's innate antioxidant, anti-inflammatory, and tissue-protecting properties may help maintain healthy cells and function of the pancreas, help fight chronic inflammation and cell damage related to insulin resistance, and work to alleviate diabetes complications. Research shows that CBD can help mend injured heart tissue and may stimulate the retina to fight inflammation leading to blindness. It may also protect against obesity: a five-year study with more than 4,000 people showed that using CBD's cousin marijuana is linked to lower levels of fasting insulin—indicating healthy insulin absorption—and to smaller waist circumference. (That means CBD may have a future in this as well.) Finally, CBD topicals have been found to soothe nerve pain and skin irritation that accompany diabetes.

DELIVERY SYSTEMS

* Ingested: capsule, sublingual tincture, concentrate, spray or drop, nano/liposomal oil, or edible for long-term inflammation and cell, tissue, and organ protection.

* Inhaled: vaporizing pen for calming immediate nerve pain and possibly promoting sleep (although it may cause wakefulness in some patients).

* Topical: salves, balms, lotions, oils, and possibly patches for diabetes-related nerve pain and skin irritation.

Digestive Issues: Heartburn (GERD); Irritable Bowel Syndrome (IBS): Diarrhea, Constipation and Hemorrhoids; Inflammatory Bowel Disease (IBD): Crohn's, Ulcerative Colitis

If you're one of the more than 40 percent of Americans who suffer from heartburn, look at triggers. Heartburn is also known as gastroesophageal disease, or GERD. The sphincter, the muscle between the esophagus and stomach, becomes lax. Instead of closing off food in the stomach where acid breaks it down, it allows a little food and acid to leak back upward into the esophagus in what's called acid reflux. To help, doctors may prescribe medications and recommend lifestyle changes: dropping spicy foods, alcohol, caffeine, chocolate, and citrus, and changing high-stress living. GERD is just one example of why it's important take care of your digestive tract, that 30-foot-long system from mouth to rectum, which includes the esophagus, stomach, and intestines and related digestive organs like the liver and pancreas. Irritable bowel syndrome (IBS) is another. This glitch in the rhythmic muscular action of the intestines produces spasms, pain, discomfort, diarrhea, and constipation. Aggravations include spicy foods, milk, wheat products, and even stress. In a 2016 issue of *Cannabis and Cannabinoid Research*, neurologist Ethan Russo proposed that IBS may be the result of a deficient ECS. Any constipation-causing conditions may also produce hemorrhoids, swollen, painful veins in the anus. In the case of autoimmune inflammatory bowl diseases (IBD) like Crohn's and ulcerative colitis, the immune system mistakes food and helpful bacteria for toxins and sends white blood cells to destroy them. Abdominal pain, diarrhea, bowel obstruction, and open sores may result. In all cases, a doctor's guidance is vital—and CBD help may be on the horizon.

WHAT CBD CAN DO: Because the GI tract is controlled by the nervous system, it is hugely affected by the endocannabinoid system and its receptors. Studies show that CBD interacts with receptors to lower inflammation linked to gastrointestinal disorders ranging from colon cancer to GERD to IBD to hemorrhoids. A 2012 study in mice with colitis by Dr. Rudolf Schicho at Austria's Medical University of Graz showed that CBD suppositories and topicals reduced inflammation and the severity of bowel disease. As of 2018, Dr. Schicho continues working toward a similar treatment for humans. Experts hold up CBD's antioxidant and cell-protective nature for soothing GERD and calming stress, which contributes to GERD; for quelling anxiety, which contributes to IBS; and for addressing side effects of IBS and IBD, such as pain and nausea (see Pain, page 112, and Nausea, page 109). CBD suppositories and bath salts help soothe hemorrhoids and fight accompanying infection.

DELIVERY SYSTEMS

* Ingested: capsule, sublingual tincture, concentrate, spray or drop, nano/liposomal oil, or edible for long-term inflammation, stress, appetite loss, and other symptoms depending on the specific kind of disorder. Avoid alcohol tinctures for any digestive disorder.

* Inhaled: vaporizing pen for immediate relief for acute symptoms such as nausea and pain.

* Topical: salves for painful or infected hemorrhoids.

Eating Disorders (Anorexia, Cachexia, Obesity)

"I need to lose weight" is a common American expression, especially after the holidays—and it's one to take seriously. Weight can be a matter of life or death, both for those who suffer from obesity and for those at the opposite end of the spectrum—fighting anorexia and cachexia. In 2015–16, the Centers for Disease Control set the number of obese Americans at 93.3 million. Besides being uncomfortable, making it hard to shop for clothes, and leading to social exclusion, obesity is downright dangerous. Heavy fat stores, especially accumulated around the abdomen, release chemicals that trigger inflammation and lead to high blood pressure, heart disease, stroke, GERD, type 2 diabetes, sleep apnea, and some kinds of cancers. That said, fat is a beautiful thing in the right amounts: it lends shape and grace to face and figure, protects bones and organs, and wraps us in insulation when cold weather calls. When a person develops an eating disorder such as anorexia and cachexia, the loss of fat also leads to a cannibalism of other body parts, like muscle, bone, skin, and even the brain. Sometimes fat remains, but muscles deteriorate. A person can literally waste away. A high percentage of people in the late stages of HIV/AIDS; cancer; tuberculosis; arthritis; liver, heart, and kidney disease; or Parkinson's and other neurodegenerative diseases can become emaciated from appetite loss. Lack of vitamin-rich food intake leads to a compromised immune system and the inability to fight other infections. Disinterest in food is often triggered by chemotherapy or other appetite-squelching drugs required to fight the primary infection. Sometimes psychological disorders are responsible: Anxiety, stress, and depression can all make even the most mouthwatering triple chocolate volcano cake a chore to behold, much less eat. And there's anorexia, often considered a teenager's curse—in which a young woman or man is a slave to staying thin, obsessing about the amount of food they eat and their body image. This can begin in childhood or later in life. There is a role for CBD and its cousin cannabinoids in helping regulate food intake. At the end of the day, nutritious food is key to healing.

WHAT CBD CAN DO: Deanna Gabriel Vierck says: "Triggers for many eating disorders are emotional: anxiety, depression, trauma, and stress [see

Anxiety, Stress, and Depression, pages 67–69]. Hemp's ability to address these roots has a big effect on eating disorders." Studies with cannabis show that it operates on these other levels, too: First, as a digestive aid (see Digestive Issues, page 87). Second, to help ease nausea and vomiting (see Nausea and Vomiting, page 109). Third, to help control appetite—either by stimulating it in undereaters or suppressing it in overeaters. The last point seems contradictory, but studies are showing that cannabinoids may interact with the endocannabinoid system's CB1 receptor to stimulate appetite by enhancing the desire for food and increasing the sense of reward a person gets from food intake. On the other hand, cannabinoids may interact with the same receptors to decrease an overweight person's constant appetite. How? One theory is that cannabinoids have a bidirectional effect; that is, they adapt differently to different body chemistries to effect the needed change. Patients with late-stage diseases especially benefit from the appetite enhancement, since the disease itself, especially in conjunction with chemotherapy and other drugs to treat the disease, dampens healthy hunger pangs.

DELIVERY SYSTEMS

* Ingested: capsule, sublingual tincture, concentrate, spray or drop, or nano/liposomal oil to increase or decrease appetite and address nausea; adding hemp seed oil rich in omega-3s may help in stimulation.

* Inhaled: vaporizing pen to quickly stimulate or slow appetite.

Endocrine Disorders

If your endocrine system is having a bad, day, you'll know it. Working with its staunch ally the endocannabinoid system, the endocrine system is all about regulating your hormones—and as any woman in menopause knows, hormone imbalance can mean roller-coaster days. The endocrine system is a series of glands, with supporting organs, that release hormones into the bloodstream to guide and balance basic body processes: heartbeat, bone and tissue growth, conception, and so much more. This massive system includes these key glands: the thymus, which helps form the immune system in children; the thyroid, which controls metabolism; the parathyroid, which triggers bone development; the pineal, which helps you sleep; the adrenal, which releases cortisol to relieve stress and shore up metabolism and immune function; and the male testes, which release sex hormones and sperm. An umbrella "master gland," the pituitary, actually controls thyroid and other glands, triggering puberty and keeping bone growth, menstruation, and breast milk production on schedule. Organs play a part, too: The brain area called the hypothalamus tells the adrenal and pituitary glands when to produce hormones to do their respective jobs; the pancreas sends out insulin, keeping you diabetes-free; and the female ovaries release sex hormones and eggs. An endocrine disorder develops when too little or too much of a hormone is released—perhaps because of genetic inheritance, disease, a tumor, or medication. In the United States, diabetes is the most common endocrine disturbance (see Diabetes, page 86). Other imbalances may prompt hyper- or hypothyroidism or infertility. Often one imbalance will trigger another, creating a domino effect. If you're feeling continual fatigue and weakness, see a health care professional right away. Your next stop may be a specialist called an endocrinologist, who'll help you determine treatment steps. In the meantime, look at CBD's potential.

WHAT CBD CAN DO: Research shows a definite link between the endocannabinoid system and the endocrine system and their roles in homeostasis. CBD has been shown to support CB1 receptors in the brain and nervous system and CB2 receptors in the immune system (see Immune System Enhancement, page 00), to enhance endocrine function. Research published in the journal *Endocrine-Related Cancer* holds that endocannabinoids in a healthy, toned ECS appear to halt the growth of cancer cells in the thyroid, breast, and prostate. In addition, a healthy ECS helps balance weight, enhance energy, and build bones—all linked to the endocrine system. Type 2 diabetes patients had hopeful news after a study published in 2017 in *Cannabis and Cannabinoid Research* reported that CBD helped lower production of the hormone resistin, linked to obesity and insulin resistance. In the realm of fertility, studies show that CB1 receptors populate the ovaries and the lining of the uterus, and the endocannabinoid called anandamide helps the fertilized egg implant and grow. Testing continues on the role and safety of CBD and other cannabinoids taken for and during pregnancy; always consult a health care professional.

DELIVERY SYSTEMS

* Ingested: capsule, sublingual tincture, concentrate, spray or drop, nano/liposomal oil, edibles for long-term boost to endocannabinoid tone and hormone regulation through the endocrine system.

Epilepsy and Other Seizure Disorders

Epilepsy is a chronic neurological disease in which unpredictable seizures take place. These begin in the brain as a result of abnormal, overwhelming electrical signals called "storms." Storms may originate in a specific part of the brain or generally, across the brain. They are suffered by children and adults. In children, the condition may be genetic, or it may be caused by brain injury, infection, or a mother's drug use during pregnancy; in older people, Alzheimer's disease, a tumor, or stroke may be the catalyst. Sometimes seizures are a one-time event caused by fever, trauma, drug abuse, or even extreme stress. During a seizure a person may or may not retain awareness and may or may not experience uncontrollable movements. The unpredictable nature of a seizure can make for an isolated lifestyle, with constant concern: will it happen soon? More than 20 traditional drugs on the market have treated epilepsy, with such side effects as appetite loss, nausea and vomiting, fatigue, dizziness, and dependency. Only recently has Epidiolex, an exciting breakthrough drug, been approved for public use for some severe epilepsies—with great effectiveness, although it, too, has side effects to be considered. Its main ingredient? CBD.

WHAT CBD CAN DO: In June 2018, Epidiolex was approved by the U.S. Food and Drug Administration in an oral solution to treat seizures in Lennox-Gastaut syndrome and Dravet syndrome, two severe forms of epilepsy. For children two years of age and older, it is the first cannabis-based, FDA-approved drug and the first for Dravet syndrome. Use of cannabis to treat epilepsy has been recorded since the 10th century, but the need for an FDA-approved medicine was brought to light by a three-year-old. Charlotte Figi, suffering from Dravet's, could not go long without seizures that drained her and her family—sometimes 300 times a week. In 2009, Charlotte's parents worked with growers cultivating high-CBD cannabis in Colorado and with researchers who knew its profoundly calming effects to try a CBD-rich extract from the plant. Soon Charlotte was laughing and playing like any other toddler. Medical reporter Dr. Sanjay Gupta brought her story to millions across America; soon that strain of cannabis became known as Charlotte's Web. Simultaneously, a UK drug company had been developing CBD-based epilepsy medicine, and the stars aligned with rigorous testing to bring a new product to market in the U.S. in 2018, within a decade of Charlotte's experience. Longstanding trials had shown that CBD stops convulsions without causing side effects. How? Probably by interacting with CB1 and CB2 receptors—and multiple others—in the ECS to keep information flowing smoothly in the brain (disruption appears to trigger a seizure), or by protecting parts of the brain where seizures start. Researchers see promise for new medicines ahead.

DELIVERY SYSTEMS

* Ingested: capsule, sublingual tincture, concentrate, spray or drop, nano/liposomal oil, or edible for seizure control, with type and dosage depending on type of epilepsy. Glycerin, not alcohol-based tinctures, is recommended for children.

* Inhaled: vaporizing pen to control seizure are recommended for adult use only.

Eye Health and Disease

According to the National Eye Institute, by 2030 nearly 60 million Americans will suffer forms of sight loss or blindness, including cataracts, macular degeneration, retinopathy, and glaucoma. These conditions are largely age-related, so living longer is likely to mean "seeing" these on the horizon. Fortunately, cataract, a film that develops over the lens as we age or if the eye has been injured, can be removed through a brief, standard procedure that has a relatively short recovery time. Retinopathy is a complication of diabetes in which vessels in the retina—the light-sensitive tissue at the back of the eye—may swell or grow abnormally. (See Diabetes, page 86.) Macular degeneration destroys the macula, the part of the eye located in the retina that allows us to see objects clearly; chances for development skyrocket after the age of 80. In glaucoma, the flow of fluid inside the eye slows down, causing pressure to build, which gradually damages the optic nerve and destroys sight. Some diseases are genetic, and others are unstoppable as we age and experience the regular wear and tear of life. Good practices can help keep your eyes healthy and sight clear for decades: shield them from bright sun; if you wear eye makeup, clean it off thoroughly each night; keep blood vessels healthy and circulation in tip-top shape by exercising every day and eating a diet filled with vitamins and omega-3-rich fish, nuts, fruits, and vegetables. The brighter the fruit and veggie colors (red peppers, orange carrots, deep green spinach), the more packed with eye-protective vitamins A, C, and E they are. CBD is moving in to help.

WHAT CBD CAN DO: The endocannabinoid system plays a major part in eye health, via CB1 and CB2 receptors. An NIH-supported study in a 2018 issue of *Cannabis and Cannabinoid Research* underscores that CBD, along with THC, interacts with these receptors to reduce the pain and inflammation from surface eye injury that leads to cataracts. Other studies have shown that CBD and THC can help reduce small rips in the retina that trigger macular degeneration and that THC helps reduce the pressure buildup that causes glaucoma. CBD and THC both have neuroprotective properties; that is, they help protect cells from damage and guard those already damaged from devolving into chronic disease. While patients taking oral forms have reported eye improvement for near- or far-sightedness, eye drops and sprays for glaucoma and other diseases are still being tested and show promise.

DELIVERY SYSTEMS

* Ingested: capsule, sublingual tincture, concentrate, spray or drop, nano/liposomal oil, or edible for lowering long-term inflammation, high blood pressure, anxiety, and aiding retinal and blood vessel health.

Fibromyalgia

A dull, body-wide ache in muscle and bone, sleepless nights, exhausted days, forgetfulness, and bad mood: they're all symptoms of this intangible disease. Where does it come from? Symptoms may be triggered by the trauma of a car accident, the psychological stress of a rocky marriage, a low-grade infection, or invasive surgery. The residual physical or psychological pain builds up over time. Research shows that such an accumulation can stimulate nerves and change the brain. Not only does the brain release more chemicals that signal pain, but pain receptors also remember the pain and grow more sensitive to it, so that each pain signal causes them to overreact. This leads to full-blown musculoskeletal pain. The unrelenting full-body ache may be accompanied by migraines, anxiety, depression, tempomandibular joint disorder (TMJ), irritable bowel syndrome, restless leg syndrome, and sleep apnea. You may sleep a full eight hours but awaken exhausted. And throughout the day you may find yourself in a "fibro fog"—it's almost impossible to focus and stay focused. If you're a woman, you're seven times more likely than a man to develop fibromyalgia. The condition has also been seen to run in families, suggesting a genetic link. But most often it can be traced to physical or emotional trauma or infection. Pain relievers, antidepressants, and even calming antiseizure drugs may be prescribed; and a regimen of physical therapy, including non-impact, water-based exercises, helps build flexibility and strength. Counseling to help pinpoint the source of stress and anxiety is also key. CBD would like to help.

WHAT CBD CAN DO: One theory behind fibromyalgia is that the endocannabinoid system is defective. It may produce too few or too many endocannabinoids. For instance, one endocannabinoid called anandamide, which plays a role in exercise-induced euphoria, or runner's high, may be overproduced and circulate throughout the body. While the stimulus is joyful in the right amount, too much is painful. CBD may arrest this overproduction, or it may interrupt the nerve pathways that send pain signals from the brain to the body. In addition, CBD's anti-inflammatory effect may help relieve general pain and swelling. CBD along with THC in a pharmaceutical called Sativex, in FDA testing as of 2018, was taken by more than 2,000 patients and found to help relieve fibromyalgia pain. In 2017, a 72-year-old sufferer's story in the respected online resource *Project CBD* told how the woman's own CBD juice recipe not only eased her fibromyalgia pain but also helped her withdraw from pain-reducing opiates her doctor had prescribed a decade earlier. A promising 2018 study published in the *Journal of Clinical Rheumatology* used medical cannabis (THC-rich) to treat fibromyalgia pain. Every patient recorded improvement, and half discontinued other pharmaceutical prescription. Wrote the study directors: "Very rarely as physicians have we encountered such responses in real-life medicine."

DELIVERY SYSTEMS:

* Ingested: capsule, sublingual tincture, concentrate, spray or drop, nano/liposomal oil for long-term inflammation, pain, and related anxiety and insomnia. May be enhanced by use of hemp seed oil with omega-3s.
* Inhaled: vaporizing pen to relieve pain, stress, anxiety.
* Topical: salves, balms, lotions, oils to help address pain and inflammation.

Headache and Migraine

It's been a tough day, and here it comes again: the ache radiating from neck and shoulders and face…the building discomfort that seems to hold your head in a vise. A tension headache is the icing on the day's cake. Along with the tension, it may have been aggravated by dehydration, lack of sleep, or even poor posture. It's not pleasant, but you may want to count your blessings. It is not a migraine: This severe headache can inhabit half your head with a pulsating vigor. Dizziness, nausea, facial tingling, and sensitivity to light and sound may urge you to a dark, quiet room, perhaps for a few hours, perhaps for 72 or more. Often, the throbbing begins with an aura, in which vision is interrupted by a blind spot, or flashing lights. Activity makes it worse. The single comfort is that you are not alone—some one billion people around the world suffer migraines, 38 million alone in the United States. Nor is it a cluster headache: This one concentrates around

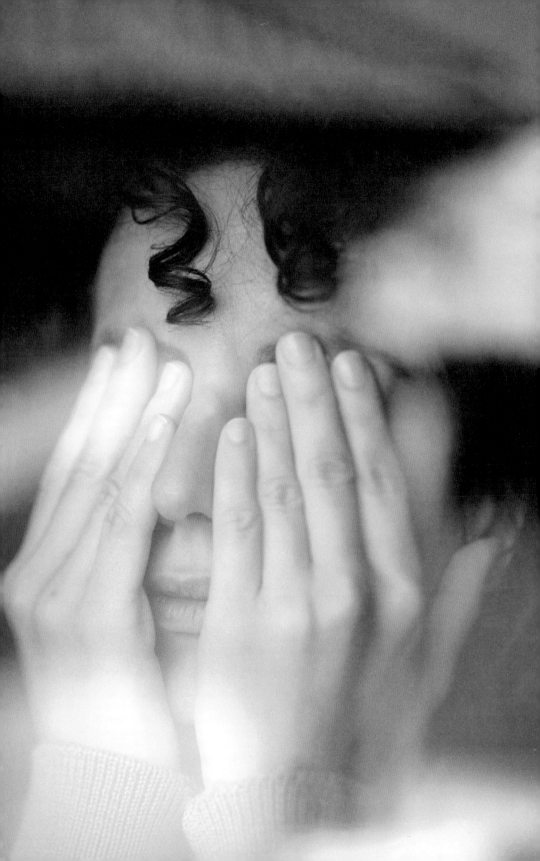

a single eye. The eye becomes watery and the nostril below it runny. As soon as it fades, it may appear again throughout the day . . . or over a few months. And then there's the sinus headache accompanying a sinus infection. It concentrates between your eyes and is complicated by a fever. And then there is the rebound headache—a reaction from a pain reliever you took to help the headache in the first place. Sometimes it seems like a no-win situation. What's happening? Research indicates that headaches may happen because of inflammation on the surface of the brain. And what do you do about it? Tension headaches—and some migraines—may resolve with over-the-counter remedies like ibuprofen and acetaminophen. Other, stronger medications are prescribed for most migraines and for cluster headaches. When it starts, try this: rest in a dark, quiet room; apply hot or cold compresses to your neck; massage your temples. Scientists have found that sipping a small amount of caffeine may help, possibly by affecting blood vessel diameter; it also helps increase the uptake of acetaminophen or other pain-relieving medicine. CBD is finding a place among the remedies.

WHAT CBD CAN DO: Research is showing that migraines may occur because of an endocannabinoid deficiency and an unusual response to inflammation. Here's the theory: A migraine may be triggered by bright lights, chemicals, premenstrual hormones, unpleasant smells, allergies, anxiety, or chronic pain disorders. If the ECS were healthy, such a trigger would cause the release of endocannabinoids to balance the system and keep pain in check. But that release doesn't seem to happen in people who suffer migraines. Instead, other chemicals flood the system, dilating blood vessels on the surface of the brain, increasing pressure and inflammation, and prompting pain. This is where CBD may help: In a 2008 issue of *Neuro Endocrinology Letters*, Dr. Ethan Russo explained that cannabinoids have been shown to "block spinal, peripheral, and gastrointestinal mechanisms that promote pain in headache, fibromyalgia, IBS and related disorders." A 2010 study in *Experimental Neurology* noted that activating the ECS with cannabinoids may be "a promising therapeutical tool" for fighting inflammation and migraine pain. And a 2017 issue of *Cannabis and Cannabinoid Research* reported that "CBD has shown efficacy for headache-related conditions"; that cannabinoids could likely stimulate the ECS and help treat the pain at its source; and that human clinical trials were a next step in potentially making cannabinoids a mainstream headache medication.

DELIVERY SYSTEMS

* Ingested: capsule, sublingual tincture, concentrate, spray or drop, nano/liposomal oil, edibles to help prevent inflammation that causes headache, or to address inflammation, pain, and nausea that accompany headache.

NOTE: First-time CBD use may cause initial headache as it detoxifies the system.

* Inhaled: vaporizing pen for acute pain and anxiety.

* Topical: salves, balms, lotions, oils to massage into temples for pain and inflammation.

Heart Health and Disease

Too many of us have lost loved ones to this deadly disease. The best thing you can do to prevent it in others you love—and yourself—is to know what it's all about. Some heart conditions, such as valve malfunction, thickening of the heart walls, or arrhythmia—an irregular heartbeat—may be genetic, caused by a virus, or the side effect from a toxin or drug. But heart, or cardiovascular (cardio: heart; vascular: veins), disease is usually caused by a single nasty process: the arteries filling up with fatty plaque. It sticks to artery walls, stiffening and blocking them so blood no longer flows smoothly and plentifully to tissues and organs—including your heart. A diet high in fat, sugar, and cholesterol; smoking; stress; lack of exercise; diabetes; and being overweight all contribute to the creation of plaque and plaque buildup. The body becomes inflamed. As blockage increases, the heart works overtime to pump enough blood to keep other parts of the body going. Blood pressure—the force needed for the blood to circulate through the veins—rises, and a person develops hypertension. Heart attack, stroke, or aneurysm may follow suddenly. Peripheral artery disease may develop, in which extremities, mostly the legs, receive too little blood flow, causing

**Maggie McLaughlin, mom on
pain, muscle spasms, headache, and pet care**

"I broke my neck 20 years ago diving into a swimming pool,"
says Maggie McLaughlin, who lives in Oregon. "The break was a
'hangman's break,' and while I am incredibly lucky to be alive and
walking, I have been dealing with pain and muscle spasms ever
since. My exploration into CBD was inspired by my desire to get
off prescription pain medication. Over a couple months I used
CBD tinctures to wean myself off Vicodin. If I could, I would
still use it daily, but at this point in time medical marijuana in
Oregon is more affordable than high-quality CBD. That said, I
do use CBD tinctures for arthritis — mostly during the winter
months when it's rainy. My daughters use it, too. One has had
hormone-related headaches since she was a teenager, suffering
each time her cycle began. At the beginning of her recent
pregnancy, the fluctuating hormones gave her terrible headaches.
She wanted as little medical intervention as possible, and when
acupuncture wasn't helping, she turned to a CBD salve with
peppermint. She massaged it into her temples and it was like a
miracle: the pain disappeared. She was floored. She used it for
her first trimester, then was fine—and her healthy baby was
delivered in December. *My other daughter gives it to her 12-year-
old dog, who suffers from anxiety and joint pain. The difference is
like night and day!*"

pain when walking. One of the key components of plaque is cholesterol—a waxy, fat-like substance that actually produces good things like vitamin D. But too much can combine with other substances in the blood to form the vein-narrowing plaque. A diet rich in fruits, vegetables, and omega-3 fish has anti-inflammatory effects and can help control high cholesterol and plaque buildup. Through his more than decade-old study titled *Blue Zones*, researcher Dan Buettner shows that heart-healthy populations are concentrated in places where diets are rich in fruits, vegetables, and fish; people work outdoors well into their 80s and after; smoking is uncommon; and lifestyle and spiritual outlook keep stress at bay. Even if you've suffered a heart attack, it's not too late to adjust your own lifestyle to prevent another. The *Blue Zones* lifestyle is a place to start. CBD has shown its worth as an inflammation fighter, too.

WHAT CBD CAN DO: Over years of research, scientists have found that CBD engages with the endocannabinoid system to reduce inflammation and oxidation in organs and systems throughout the body. A 2013 study in the *British Journal of Pharmacology* showed its role in relaxing arterial walls, helping lower plaque formation, increasing blood flow, and protecting the arteries against damage from inflammation. All these points help lower blood pressure and counteract hypertension, which leads to heart disease. Another study with more than 4,500 people showed that cannabis users had higher levels of good cholesterol (HDL); and research in the 2015 journal *Obesity* analyzed 700 Inuit cannabis users, showing both a rise in HDL and a drop in levels of bad cholesterol, or LDL. CBD is also a well-known antioxidant, which protects healthy cells from damage. Scientists see a potential role in protecting the heart from cardiomyopathy, sometime triggered by diabetes, in which the heart muscle becomes rigid so it can't pump blood efficiently through the body. Finally, hemp seed oil, which may be purchased in a health food store, is packed with heart-protective omega-3s.

DELIVERY SYSTEMS:

* Ingested: capsule, sublingual tincture, concentrate, spray or drop, nano/liposomal oil, or edible for long-term protection against inflammation and vascular damage that promotes heart disease.

Immune System Enhancement

The immune system is almighty. Without its reinforcing effects, we leave ourselves open to every possible disease, from depression to obesity. Pause for a moment and think about the world around you: jam-packed with viruses, bacteria, fungi, you name it. We all should be walking, coughing germ receptacles. Instead, humans for the most part are walking wonders, with heads held high, relying on an intensive system of organs, cells, and molecules that spring into action whenever toxins threaten. Those could be poisonous chemicals, cancer cells, disease-carrying microbes, the occasional rusty nail. In healthy children and young adults, the immune system usually operates on all signals to fight off viral and bacterial invaders. Ideally, it ignores harmless pollen, dust mites, animal dander, and our normal cells. But sometimes it doesn't. Suddenly we are allergic: sneezing when we walk outside in springtime or when the dog bounds into the room. In most severe cases, the "something wrong" is the system's turning against the body's own cells. These autoimmune diseases, such as lupus, can be life-threatening. Some of us are born with a compromised immune system; for most of us, however, it operates full force in our youth, but weakens as we age. Environmental factors can dampen it, too: chronic stress and disease may wear down its quick reaction and effectiveness; lack of sleep and a diet high in sugars and unhealthy fats can throw it off balance and trigger inflammation; medications like chemotherapy may suppress it, leaving you open to infection. If you feel that you are always fighting a cold, sinusitis, or a urinary tract, bladder, or kidney infection, you may have to look no further than your compromised immune system. Recognizing your immune system's role in your vital, thriving life is the start of a beautiful relationship that will just get better with care. Remember these key points: Sleep. Calm down. Eat well. Exercise. And never underestimate the power of a human or spiritual touch. CBD just may be an ally.

WHAT CBD CAN DO: The very anti-inflammatory nature of CBD and other plant cannabinoids sets them up to be immune system boosters. And that's just what scientists are finding out. In a 2017 *Frontiers of Immunology* article, researchers underscored that the endocannabinoid system is considered the "homeostatic 'gate-keeper' of the immune system" and that ECS receptors play a vital role in healthy immune responses. That includes fighting the inflammation that comes with generally poor health and infection. Along with their "anticonvulsive, analgesic, antiemetic, and anti inflammatory" properties, CBD and THC appear to work together with ECS cannabinoids and receptors to protect immune function. A series of animal studies with CBD—sometimes also with THC—showed support of the immune system during an organ transplant; protection of the brain after a stroke; stopping tumor growth; prevention of brain damage from meningitis; and protection of the brain against malaria. CBD was also held up as a possible treatment for post-Ebola syndrome, with its joint and muscle pain, nerve damage, and blindness.

DELIVERY SYSTEMS

* Ingested: capsule, sublingual tincture, concentrate, spray or drop, nano/liposomal oil, or edible for long-term fight against inflammation and support of immune function.

Liver Disease

A healthy liver is a major digestive aid and rids your body of toxins. But if you have been infected by a virus, have a genetic disorder, drink too much, or fight obesity, you may develop cirrhosis, or scarring, of the liver. The first symptom is that your eyes, and possibly your skin, appear yellowish or jaundiced—a sign that a chemical called bilirubin is not being processed. Inside, scarring turns the liver lumpy and hard, blocking blood flow. Toxins being carried by the blood for cleansing in the liver, like bilirubin and ammonia, now back up into the body and cause other problems, including that sallow color. Some 25,000 people across the United States die each year from liver cirrhosis caused by prescription medications like acetaminophen, exposure to other toxic chemicals, and alcohol abuse. That prompts a message to all Americans: if you even moderately consume alcohol, remember to limit yourself to one drink a day if you're a woman and two if you're a man. The most common liver virus is hepatitis—contracted through contaminated water, needles, or bodily fluids such as blood, semen, and saliva. Some 200 million people around the globe, and more than 3 million in the U.S. alone, are infected with the hepatitis C virus, the leading cause of liver failure after cirrhosis. In some cases, genetics play a part and you've inherited the disease. In other cases, an autoimmune disorder prompts the immune system to attack your healthy liver. And there is the big "C"—cancer—escape from which none of us is guaranteed. If you're traveling to certain countries or in a high-risk environment, talk to a doctor about a hepatitis vaccine. Be careful to use a condom during sex with a little-known partner, and if you're headed to a tattoo parlor, be sure it's clean. Being careless in both situations can lead to your contracting hepatitis. And finally, watch your weight and diet: obesity can lead to fatty liver, which looks a lot like one affected by alcohol—even if you've never had an alcoholic drink. CBD may have a bright future in your world.

WHAT CBD CAN DO: Research published in 2017 in *Pharmacognosy Research* suggests that CBD may interact with CB2 receptors to aid in antiviral activity, and scientists recommend further testing as a potential treatment for viral hepatitis, especially when used with existing therapies. For those who consume alcoholic beverages, CBD may be a light on the horizon: First, it has many of the liver-protectant qualities found in the milk thistle compound silymarin: It's rich in flavonoids, making it both anti-inflammatory and an antioxidant. Studies using silymarin show that it may help prevent toxins from infiltrating liver cells and from interacting with CB1 and CB2 receptors to keep the liver from developing fibrosis, which leads to toxin buildup in the body. Second, an animal study published in a 2017 *Scientific Reports* found that CBD helped arrest liver injury caused by alcohol, possibly by blocking inflammation. It also suggested CBD's "therapeutic potential" for alcohol-related liver diseases based on inflammation, oxidation, and fatty liver. A human trial may be coming soon.

DELIVERY METHOD

* Ingested: capsule, sublingual tincture, concentrate, spray or drop, nano/ liposomal oil, edibles to protect against inflammation and cell damage.

Lyme Disease

After a day hiking in the woods, you feel refreshed and relaxed. Then you look down at your arm and notice a dot that shouldn't be there. Looking closer, you see it's a tick. Pull it out quickly—with care. Keep it in a closed jar, and then watch the bite area over the next few days. If a bull's eye–shaped rash appears, you've likely been infected by a black-legged, or deer, tick—*Ixodes scapularis*. These tiny invaders—just bigger than a poppy seed—can be identified by black legs and a roundish black pattern on their back. As they feast on blood of other mammals, including deer, they pick up a certain spiral-shaped bacterium, *Borrelia bergdorferi*, which can be transferred when a tick attaches to you. If removed within 36 hours, a tick often has not had time to transmit disease; after that, a different story can unfold. Over a period of months or years, infection can bring chronic joint, nervous system, and heart problems. Stay watchful: if flu-like symptoms appear, including chills and fever, see a health care professional to determine next steps. Lyme disease is often overdiagnosed, and you don't want to begin pumping unneeded antibiotics into your body, but caution is always the best route. The CDC reports about 30,000 cases a year—although there may be as many as 300,000 across the U.S. When outdoors, use insect repellent and cover yourself completely. Back inside, do a tick check in hard-to-see places like the groin, scalp, and armpits. Oral antibiotics can successfully treat the tick-borne bacteria, and some experts recommend bacteria-fighting licorice and garlic or immune-boosting echinacea or CBD to support them.

WHAT CBD CAN DO: While CBD has yet to be studied through medical trials for treating Lyme disease, it has been held up as a treatment for the bacterial infection (see Bacterial Infections, page 72), inflammation, and pain that accompany Lyme disease (see Inflammation, page 62, and Chronic Pain, page 112). A 2012 *Journal of Experimental Medicine* study supports its potential to "suppress chronic inflammatory and neuropathic pain." It also protects the nervous system (see Neurodegenerative Diseases, page 110) and eases the anxiety that many report feeling with the disease (see Anxiety, page 67). A study in the 2009 *Journal of Natural Products* showed that many cannabinoids have the potential to guard against tick-borne and other insect bacteria. On the education and research site Lymedisease.org, Denver physician Dr. Daniel A. Kinderlehrer notes, "The analgesic, anti-inflammatory and neuroprotective properties of cannabis make it extremely valuable as an adjunct to the treatment of tick-borne diseases."

* Ingested: capsule, sublingual tincture, concentrate, spray or drop, nano/liposomal oil, or edible for bacterial infection and long-term fight against pain and inflammation.

* Inhaled: vaporizing pen for acute anxiety and pain.

* Topical: salves, balms, lotions, oils for pain.

TIP: Pull a tick from your skin by grasping its head—not its body—with tweezers and pulling it steadily upward. Grabbing the body risks leaving tick parts behind. Clean with alcohol.

Metabolic Syndrome

This unwelcome condition is actually a cluster of simultaneous conditions: increased fat around the waist, a jump in blood sugar, exceptionally high cholesterol and triglyceride (natural fat) levels, and blood pressure that shoots through the roof. The combination puts you at risk for diabetes, heart disease, and stroke. Even though one condition alone doesn't mean you have metabolic syndrome, it does mean that you are open to serious disease— either single or combined—if you don't act quickly. First, check your waist: Is it growing larger by leaps and bounds? Is it apple-shaped rather than pear-shaped? If your fat particularly accumulates around the abdomen instead of the buttocks, legs, shoulders, or other body parts, you are prone to metabolic syndrome. Next, have your vitals checked to be sure that the other symptoms aren't waiting in the wings. You may find that your blood sugar is unusually elevated. That could signal the start of diabetes, in which cells are unable to take in sugar from the blood to use as fuel; instead, sugar builds up dangerously in the blood. (See Diabetes, page 86.) Blurry vision, fatigue, and increased thirst and urination all are symptoms. Check cholesterol and triglycerides next (see Heart Health and Disease, page 99). Are your LDL (bad cholesterol) and triglyceride numbers sky high, while HDL (good cholesterol) goes wanting? That means fatty deposits are building up in your arteries, narrowing them and causing blood to work harder to circulate through them. Blood pressure rises and, if it's left unchecked, arteries may block completely, and you'll suffer a heart attack or stroke. How vulnerable are you to developing metabolic syndrome? As you age, your susceptibility rises; and if you easily gain weight around your abdomen, keep careful watch. A family history of type 2 diabetes is a warning signal, as is your own history of heart or liver disease. Through exercise and a plant-based Mediterranean diet, you can begin right away to control weight, cholesterol and triglycerides, and blood pressure (see Eating Disorders, page 89). Start by taking a good look in the mirror, and don't wince. This beauty contest goes beyond looks— you're competing against time for a body so beautifully healthy that it will carry you into decades to come.

WHAT CBD CAN DO: Studies show that when the endocannabinoid system loses tone, it can contribute to obesity, high cholesterol, heart disease, and type 2 diabetes. Research published in the 2011 *Handbook of Experimental Pharmacology* found that CBD can help stabilize these components of metabolic disorder; it also noted the CBD appeared to slow cell damage in type 1 diabetes (see Diabetes, page 86). A 2011 study in Hungary found that CBD had the potential to interact with the hypothalamus when injury to that part of the brain triggered abnormal overeating. CBD helped shut down cravings without the side effects of pharmaceuticals. The study also found that CBD in conjunction with other therapies interacted with the immune system to help slow damage to arteries caused by high levels of glucose, or sugar, in the blood. (See the individual conditions that make up metabolic syndrome to find out more about their potential future with CBD.)

DELIVERY SYSTEMS

* Ingested: capsule, sublingual tincture, concentrate, spray or drop, nano/ liposomal oil, edibles to boost endocannabinoid tone, protect cells and arteries, and keep eating in check.

Multiple Sclerosis (MS) and Spasticity

This mysterious and devastating disease generally attacks a person between the ages of 15 and 60, affecting twice as many women as men. Autoimmune in nature, multiple sclerosis, or MS, sets in as the immune system mistakenly attacks healthy nerve fibers in the body, breaking down their protective fatty coating, called the myelin sheath. As a result, nerve impulses from the brain are slowed or blocked, and communication between the brain and body breaks down. Eventually, nerves may become permanently damaged. Mild-MS patients may experience stiffness, fatigue, dizziness, and numbness; more severe MS sufferers may lose the ability to walk as spasticity—lack of muscle control and flexibility—sets in. Tremors, facial pain, slurred speech, incontinence, and double vision or vision loss can come at any stage. What triggers the autoimmune action that prompts MS? Scientists aren't sure, but patterns suggest that both family history and the environment play a part. Those of northern European descent or living in cool climates like the northern United States and Canada may be candidates. The disease is generally "relapsing-remitting": symptoms appear and then dissipate in cycles. While there is no cure for MS, physical therapy and other treatments can step up recovery after a relapse, lifting mood, improving the immune system, and strengthening weakened muscles. Keeping the body cool is key, since heat exacerbates symptoms. The Mayo Clinic recommends a diet rich in vitamins, minerals, and plant-based omega-3 fats; watching weight; and avoiding alcohol, which impedes balance. On the horizon, a new CBD-THC treatment is making a name for itself.

WHAT CBD CAN DO: Still to be approved by the FDA, Sativex is a drug now used in European and other nations to treat MS. Sativex has a 1:1 CBD to THC ratio and is used mainly as an oral spray. Research in a 2012 issue of *Expert Review of Neurotherapeutics* held that after use, patients reported reduced spasticity and better quality of life. Since then, multiple studies support the idea that a well-toned ECS is key to regulating the nervous system and the effects of MS. Ingesting CBD and THC may stimulate endocannabinoid production to fill that void. CBD and THC may also stimulate ECS receptors to deliver anti-inflammatory, nerve-protecting, and pain-relieving properties. In a 2018 *Frontiers in Neurology* article, researchers wrote that CBD supplementation may help "reduce fatigue, pain, spasticity, and ultimately improve mobility." "Supplementation" is the key word. Talk with your health care provider about how any supplement could interact with MS medications. And ask about CBD's relative, hemp seed oil. In a study reported in the 2018 *Neuropsychiatric Disease and Treatment* journal, MS patients who used the oil reported pain and fatigue relief and increase in cognitive function and overall quality of life.

DELIVERY SYSTEMS

* Ingested: capsule, sublingual tincture, concentrate, spray or drop, nano/liposomal oil, edible to help address long-term inflammation and fatigue, and relax muscles; additional use of hemp seed oil may have anti-inflammatory benefit.
* Inhaled: vaporizing pen to address acute pain.
* Topical: salves, balms, lotions, oils for pain and circulation.

Nausea and Vomiting (Includes Motion Sickness and Pregnancy)

Even though the purpose of nausea and vomiting is to tell us something's not right or to cleanse our body of toxins, they're among our most miserable experiences. For generally healthy people, nausea and vomiting may act as a janitor, cleaning out the system during a bout of flu or food poisoning. They can be the nag reminding you that your body can't find balance as you ride in a car on a winding road. And they can be the spoiler for pregnancy joy: morning sickness signals your body's accommodation of an "invader." Chemotherapy used in cancer is another trigger for nausea; while targeting cancer cells, the drug cocktail delivers nausea as a side effect. Use of opioid drugs also can cause nausea and vomiting, as can withdrawal from them. Often, your body may need to vomit. If that's the case, drink clear liquids to restore hydration, preferably sports drinks or other fluids that also restore lost salt. Nausea can be quelled through natural remedies such as chewing ginger or sipping ginger tea. CBD offers another way.

WHAT CBD CAN DO: As early as the mid-1970s, researchers began exploring cannabis products to address the nausea and vomiting that accompanies chemotherapy. First trying THC, scientists found that it interacted with the endocannabinoid system's CB1 receptors—in the brain, gastrointestinal tract, and inner ear—to reduce the unwanted effects. More recent research finds that CBD may help stabilize the off-beat feeling through 5HT1 receptors. One explanation is that it may block nausea-prompting serotonin released by these receptors. Sufferers of chronic nausea may be anxiety-ridden, knowing what's just around the corner. That, in turn, becomes one more trigger. In these cases, studies show that CBD helps with the release of serotonin to deliver a calming, antianxiety force. (See Anxiety, page 67.)

DELIVERY SYSTEMS

* Ingested: capsule, sublingual tincture, concentrate, spray or drop, or nano/liposomal oil to ease symptoms of nausea. Capsules and edibles may be harder to intake if any kind of solid causes a nauseous reaction.

* Inhaled: vaporizing pen to quickly ease acute symptoms.

Neurodegenerative Diseases

A neurodegenerative disease begins in the brain. For unexplained reasons, neurons, or nerve cells, in the area called the basal ganglia degenerate; the production of dopamine, a chemical that aids in the transmission of nerve impulses, is reduced; and gradually symptoms set in. Unlike other cells, neurons don't reproduce, so once they are damaged or die, a person loses motor and mental function. Parkinson's, Alzheimer's, or Huntington's may follow. Symptoms for Parkinson's begin with lack of muscle control. A person may feel a tremor in a hand, which may progress to both hands, and then to their arms, legs, and head. While it may run in families, it may also be the result of environmental toxins or a severe disease like encephalitis. As it progresses, it may be accompanied by dementia. Alzheimer's is America's most common form of dementia, or memory impairment. As brain cells die, memory and mental function, such as organization, reasoning, and knowledge of how to perform daily tasks, go with them. Mood swings, depression, and aggression can accompany this state. A family history of Alzheimer's and environmental factors may also play a part in this disease. Scientists especially notice that two things—a buildup of plaque called beta-amyloid and a scrambling of proteins called tau—destroy cells and inhibit transmission of nerve impulses. Huntington's is considered a young person's disease, with symptoms often showing between ages 30 and 50. The disease is caused by an inherited defect in a single gene. As nerve cells break down, a person may suffer writhing or jerking motions or sudden outbursts. Communicating, reasoning, remembering, and performing simple tasks become challenging. Isolation, depression, and suicidal thoughts may develop. For each of these diseases, certain medicines can help control symptoms and slow progression, but there is no cure. Scientists believe that inflammation may play a key role in degeneration. Taking measures to maintain brain health can only help boost one's ability to hold them off for as long as possible and to face them with strong reserves if and when they arrive. Exercise, which boosts circulation to the brain, is key. Nutrient-rich fruits and vegetables protect brain cells with their anti-inflammatory and antioxidant powers. Omega-3 fats are abundant in brain cell membranes and can be boosted by consuming fish and olive oil. CBD can be part of the plan.

WHAT CBD CAN DO: CBD and other cannabinoids may help with these disorders because of their inherent neuroprotectant properties. CBD's anti-inflammatory and antioxidant properties may help prevent damage and degeneration in the first place. Research shows that CBD may or may not act through the endocannabinoid system to deliver its benefits for these diseases, but it appears to be working—and as of 2018 scientists are looking for the mechanism. NIH-supported studies in 2012 and 2014 showed that CBD helped reverse cognitive decline in rats treated with iron—known for triggering memory loss and present in the brains of both Parkinson's and Alzheimer's sufferers. It also helped clean out accumulated proteins and other particles that can trigger cell death. And Parkinson's patients in a 2014 trial reported improved quality of life and relief of tremors and other symptoms after a course of CBD. Finally, in a four-week trial, CBD showed promise for arresting Parkinson's-related psychosis. As of 2018, research using the potential new drug Sativex—a combination of CBD and THC—and other cannabinoid combinations shows promise for taming uncontrollable movements in Huntington's patients.

* Ingested: capsule, sublingual tincture, concentrate, spray or drop, nano/liposomal oil for stress and anxiety and long-term neuroprotective, anti-inflammatory, memory, and immune system benefits.

Pain and Chronic Pain

As with inflammation, there are two kinds of pain: acute (specific) or neuropathic (chronic). Both kinds not only bring discomfort, but they also compromise quality of life and damage tissue, leading to deeper illness. For many people, pain is an occasional and discrete event: a cut or broken arm in an accident while playing, a finger closed in a door, a sunburn. You may feel pain during an illness or after surgery. As we age, simple wear and tear may bring us chronic back and muscle aches or fingers swollen with arthritis. And certain conditions can take hold at any time, bringing chronic pain: migraine, irritable bowel syndrome, multiple sclerosis, and cancer, to name a few. It all starts with your spinal cord and brain, where the complex signaling between nerves can be interrupted by any number of daily events and conditions. In simplest terms, pain happens when a nerve ending is stimulated, perhaps by a cut and tissue damage. In more complex cases, pain results from system-wide damage to nerves, with disruption of their normal signaling—perhaps the result of an old injury or a chronic disease. Each person's experience with pain is unique. While one may take arthritis pain for granted and move through the day with a determined limp, another may be laid low by a throbbing migraine and need to lie in a dark room for 72 hours. Pain is personal, too, involving our own learning experiences and the memory of how we've reacted to pain episodes in the past. Chronic pain can bring depression and social isolation, creating more pain in a vicious cycle. The first step in treating pain is identifying how it affects you. Basic pain medications—whether over the counter or prescriptive—may well cut to the chase, but integrative practices like physical therapy, exercise, and diet are key to healing in many cases. And reach out if you're struggling—to family, friends, a trusted therapist. (See Depression, page 69.) Your health care professional is there to guide you. In the meantime, consider the potential power of CBD.

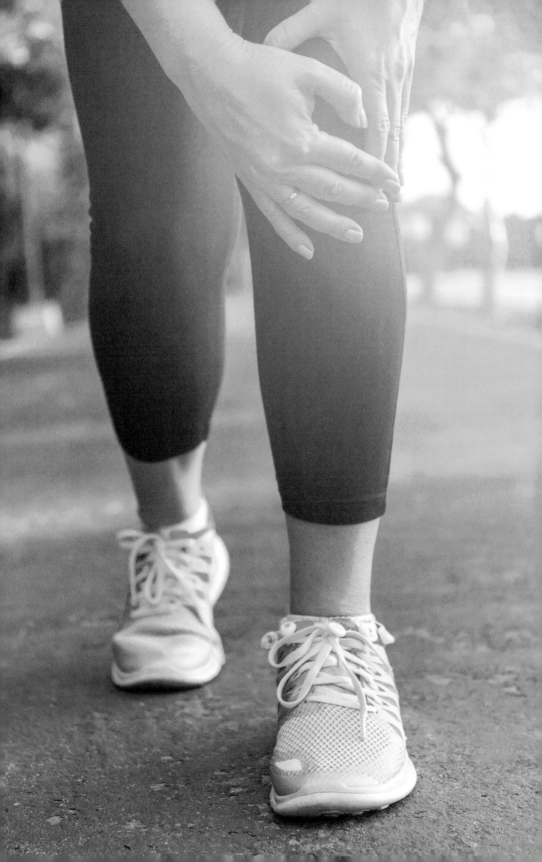

WHAT CBD CAN DO: Pain relief is the most time-honored use of the cannabis plant: it was held up as a "tonic" in China more than 4,000 years ago. A deeper scientific dive shows the potential for its cannabinoids CBD and THC to treat pain in fibromyalgia and migraine, arthritis, cancer, MS, and more. The key lies in their interaction with the ECS. Trials have shown their role in boosting the production and activity of key endocannabinoids and other chemicals in the ECS to target pain. (See Fibromyalgia, page 95, and Headache and Migraine, page 96.) For patients taking opioids for severe pain, cannabinoids may increase opioid effectiveness, which in turn can help lower the opioid dose—and also aid in withdrawal as they heal. A 2018 *Journal of Pain Research* study showed that a CBD-THC combination—present in the drug Sativex, in FDA trial as of 2018—delivered significant relief for sufferers of cancer, MS, and other pain-intensive diseases. Other cannabis plant compounds may play supporting roles: in his 2008 report in *Clinical Risk Management*, Dr. Ethan Russo noted that the terpene myrcene is both analgesic and anti-inflammatory, and that at least one flavonol has the potential to relieve pain more effectively than aspirin.

DELIVERY SYSTEMS

* Ingested: capsule, sublingual tincture, concentrate, spray or drop, nano/liposomal oil for long-term pain and inflammation control; may also help insomnia (although CBD can cause wakefulness in some people).

* Inhaled: vaporizing pen for acute pain relief.

* Topical: salves, balms, lotions, oils for back, arthritic joints, and other localized pain.

Palliative Care

As we approach the end of life, we all wish to take our leave painlessly and with serenity. Palliative care is a step in that direction. Often called hospice care, palliative care may take place in a patient's home or in a care facility, hospital, or inpatient hospice. A team made up of medical, social, and spiritual caregivers helps the patient address the many factors that can make this period one of pain and apprehension. Rather than actively trying to heal a condition, the focus is on managing pain and comfort and bringing emotional, psychological, and spiritual contentment. End-stage conditions can include cancer, congestive heart failure, pulmonary fibrosis, kidney disease, Parkinson's, Alzheimer's, and many more. In each one, pain management is key, especially with end-stage cancer. But other physical concerns, like shortness of breath, constipation, and nausea, must be managed, too. And psychological and spiritual concerns need to be addressed. Nearing the unknown can bring stress, loneliness, depression, and sleepless nights. Hospice patients often suffer anxiety as they worry about the future of their loved ones. An excellent palliative team digs deep: they help a person feel more in control by listening to personal goals;

reviewing treatment options; and keeping each team member, family members, and the patient informed along the way. While prescriptive pain medication is continued, so are steps toward emotional and spiritual peace. CBD and THC have been playing key roles in this story.

WHAT CBD CAN DO: Cannabinoids have likely been an agent for palliative care for centuries, well before the first known recorded use by cannabis pioneer Dr. William O'Shaughnessy: in 1838 he treated a patient with end-stage rabies. The doctor found that cannabis calmed the patient's violent seizures and helped him sleep until the end. A 2016 issue of *Current Oncology* reported success in using cannabis for palliative cancer care, and the author predicted that its use "will only grow with time as knowledge and acceptance become mainstream once more, as in 19th and 20th century North America and Europe." Work with end-stage patients has shown CBD and THC to tame the nausea and vomiting, among other conditions, that accompany cancer and chemotherapy. (See Nausea and Vomiting, page 109.) And, equally important, CBD is seen to improve quality of life: A 2017 study in Israel showed that cannabinoids stimulated appetite and helped patients gain weight, sleep better, and feel happier and more energized. Itching and pain were relieved, and opioid use was lower. CBD has been shown to be especially effective in lowering stress-related anxiety, likely by working with ECS receptors in the brain to reduce emotional memories linked to stressful situations. THC has been found to be the stronger medicine for pain relief and to deliver a sense of well-being, sometimes called euphoria, that helps ease patients toward the finish line.

DELIVERY METHODS:

* Ingested: capsule, sublingual tincture, concentrate, spray or drop, nano/liposomal oil, edibles for supporting quality of life: anxiety relief and general calming, nausea control, weight stabilization.

* Inhaled: vaporizing pen for relaxation and to address acute anxiety, stress, and pain.

* Topical: salves, balms, lotions, oils to relieve itching and topical pain such as arthritis or nerve pain; soothing massage to relax and relieve anxiety.

Post-Traumatic Stress (PTS)

About 10 percent of the population experience post-traumatic stress. It does not have to be triggered by being at war, although this is by far the most significant origin. Experiencing or witnessing any terrifying event is enough to bring it on—a car accident, sexual abuse, loss of a home during a fire or hurricane. Once going through such an event, a person can suffer extreme anxiety, nightmares, and frequent flashbacks. Insomnia, trouble concentrating, and being easily angered or startled are other symptoms. These may become more intense when a person is stressed or a sensory trigger brings everything flooding back: perhaps a car backfiring sends a veteran "back to war." Or the smell of a campfire triggers memories of a devastating house fire. In many cases, the mind will ease with time and distance. The exact mechanism for developing PTS is unknown, but it may have roots in the part of the brain called the amygdala, which helps process emotions and is linked to fear response. Brain scans have shown that the amygdala changes in people with PTS, resulting in heightened fear response to events, photographs, or other stimuli that remind them of the trauma. Other factors can increase a person's potential for developing PTS: the length and intensity of the experience; a previous traumatic episode; work that puts you in harm's way, such as police work or the military; inherent anxiety, depression, or guilt; substance abuse. If symptoms are severe or continue for more than a month, ruining the quality of life or bringing suicidal thoughts, it's vital that a person seek treatment. Timing is everything. The sooner you recognize the recurrent problem, the sooner you can reach out to a physical doctor, psychiatric therapist, spiritual leader, support group, or all of the above. Alcohol and drug use has been the first line of self-treatment for many veterans, but that has only made the suffering worse. CBD is showing a positive effect.

WHAT CBD CAN DO: Besides changes in the amygdala, changes in the ECS are also common for PTS sufferers. That's because so many ECS receptors are present in the amygdala and other parts of the brain involved in memory and in fear response. In PTS sufferers, ECS receptors are fewer and the endocannabinoids—which interact with them to keep the body balanced— are lower. Research has shown that CBD may interact with the ECS receptors and the entire system to help calm PTS symptoms such as stress and anxiety. (See Stress, page 63, and Anxiety, page 67.) Specifically, it has been shown to work with CB1 receptors to help expunge terrible recurring memories of an event that may lead to continual anxiety and frequent nightmares. A study in the 2017 *British Journal of Pharmacology* explained that it shows signs of disrupting the amygdala's association with fear.

DELIVERY SYSTEMS

* Ingested: capsule, sublingual tincture, concentrate, spray or drop, nano/liposomal oil to relieve anxiety, lift mood, and possibly dissipate fear memory; may also alleviate insomnia. (CBD can cause wakefulness in some people.)
* Inhaled: vaporizing pen for acute anxiety.

Prostate Health

If you are one of the 30 million men who suffer from prostate condition, you know the discomfort that comes with inflammation and painful urination. Situated just below the bladder, the prostate is a small walnut-sized gland that encircles the urethra, the tube that carries urine from the bladder to the penis. The gland also plays a part in semen buildup and ejaculation. When the prostate becomes inflamed and enlarged, it blocks the flow of urine, causing urgency and increasing the risk of bladder infection. Semen is difficult to eject. Most prostate disorders appear as a man approaches the age of 50 and beyond, but they can also happen earlier. In bacterial prostatitis, inflammation sets in as bacteria infiltrates the prostate gland. Frequent, painful urination; pain behind the testicles; lower back pain; and flu-like fatigue, fever, and chills can accompany it. Regular prostatitis, which is enlargement without bacterial infection, carries the same symptoms of frequent, painful urination and painful ejaculation, but without the flu-like symptoms. Older men are the targets for benign prostatic hyperplasia (BPH), which usually sets in between the ages of 50 and 60; beyond the age of 80 there is a 90 percent chance of developing it. Unlike the infected prostate, this one simply enlarges so much that urine can no longer flow smoothly. Growth may be prompted by a change in hormones, much like

TESTIMONIAL

**Ben Cardamone, Vietnam War veteran,
Warrior StoryField Project volunteer on
post-traumatic stress**

"I was in Viet Nam in 1968–69 as a Marine Corps medevac crew chief on a helicopter," says Ben Cardamone. "It was horrific—handling the dead and wounded, cleaning out the bloody cargo hold each time. I came home pretty crazy. I moved outside Boulder, Colorado, and just checked out. At first I started meditation and yoga to help calm my anxiety. Like all my other friends, I had been smoking pot since I'd been in Viet Nam. But there was something about the cannabis plant that made me believe there was more to it than just smoking it. About 35 years ago, I experimented with using a hemp-based CBD tincture. It had no psychoactive effect, but I could feel that it was doing something good for my body. Gradually I realized that it was also helping me find clarity that I hadn't experienced in a long while. I could see a way forward; and I was less anxious. In addition, I changed my lifestyle. I've been a vegetarian since the war—almost 50 years now—and so I have to give credit in part to a holistic lifestyle of eating well, meditating, and yoga. But CBD definitely plays a big part. Until a few years ago, I still consumed a moderate amount of alcohol, but I've stopped that, too. *Now I use a CBD salve to rub into an old shoulder wound from the war, and a couple drops of nano/liposomal oil in the morning and at night. I feel the CBD effect even more—and I feel even better.* I'm 72 now, and the same weight as when I joined the Marine Corps. And I don't take any pharmaceuticals. I work every day to introduce the healing powers of CBD to other vets, old and young."

the one women go through during menopause. This increases production of a compound called dihydrotestosterone (DHT), which in turn causes cells to multiply until the prostate blocks the urethra's path. A weak urine stream is accompanied by frequency and urgency, but inability to begin the flow—and to stop it; at last, the bladder may not fully empty, leading to bladder infection. Finally, there is cancer. Prostate cancer is one of the most common cancers in men; many will get it just by living long enough. Simply, cells become abnormal and gradually grow into a tumor. Usually it grows slowly and is harmless while concentrated in the prostate gland; but others can grow quickly and eventually metastasize, or move to other parts of the body. The signs are similar to the other signs of prostate dysfunction, along with pelvic pain and blood in the urine. Always see a health care professional when you see these signs. Bacterial prostatitis may be treated with antibiotics. Noninfectious prostatitis has been treated with muscle relaxants, hot baths, and physical therapy for relaxation while urinating. Prescription medications and sometimes surgery may alleviate BPH. Maintaining healthy weight through exercise and diet and consuming antioxidant-rich fruits and vegetables helps maintain prostate health naturally. An herb called saw palmetto has also been touted for prostate health. CBD has shown benefits, too.

WHAT CBD CAN DO: A 2014 study published in *Pharmacology and Pharmacy* specifically on CBD and prostate cancer found that CBD is anti-inflammatory and may interact with the ECS receptors to inhibit the growth of cancer cells. It noted that CBD may "inhibit spheroid formation," the abnormal shape a cell can take when it turns cancerous. As an anti-inflammatory, studies show it likely inhibits the action of cells that boost inflammation and supports cells that halt inflammation. Such action has been seen to relieve both kinds of prostatitis. Also, CBD's antibacterial properties may fight infectious prostatitis. (See Antibiotic-Resistant Bacterial Infection, page 72.) In addition, CBD's properties may help control pain, promote bladder health, and ease the anxiety and depression related to the condition (see Pain and Chronic Pain, page 112, Bladder Health and Incontinence, page 80, Anxiety, page 67, and Depression, page 69.)

* Ingested: capsule, sublingual tincture, concentrate, spray or drop, nano/liposomal oil, or food to work against long-term inflammation, cell damage, cancer growth; to help address bacterial infection, pain, anxiety, and depression accompanying disease.

* Inhaled: vaporizing pen for acute anxiety.

Psychological Disorders: Schizophrenia, Bipolar Disorder, Mood Disorder

These are dark concerns, but with treatment there is light. Schizophrenia is a serious disorder in which daily reality becomes distorted. A person's thoughts and speech may be jumbled, and he or she may experience audible and visual hallucinations; irrational actions; delusional thoughts such as paranoia; and a sliding scale of emotions. Agitation, depression, resistance to instructions, no reaction or overreaction to a conversation or event, bizarre or inappropriate postures—all of these impair daily activities. Ultimately, it's impossible to function. Schizophrenia is an incurable, chronic condition that sentences a person to lifelong treatment. While symptoms can be controlled and may even go into remission over time, they always remain present below the surface. In teenagers the symptoms may be concurrent with the usual withdrawal, lack of motivation, and irritability of that age, making it harder to diagnose; but visual hallucinations are a sure sign. Experts believe that schizophrenia is likely the result of some combination of family history, brain chemistry, environmental events, or drug use at an early age. Triggers may include birth complications, brain injury, exposure to chemicals, a neurodegenerative disease like Parkinson's, or even a father's older age at time of conception. If someone you love appears to be suffering from schizophrenia, work with a health care professional immediately to determine treatment, which may include hospitalization. If not kept under control, symptoms may lead to depression, social isolation, health and financial problems, homelessness, and even suicide.

Bipolar disorder, affects only 2 to 3 percent of the global population. According to the National Institutes of Health, its signals are "clear changes in mood, energy, and activity levels"—from being extremely "up," or manic, to extremely "down," or depressed. Mood swings can happen rarely or several times a year, triggered by high stress or trauma—like the death of a loved one—and affect sleep, activity, judgment, and behavior. As with schizophrenia, genetics often plays a part, and diagnosis in teenagers tends to be harder because the actions mirror teenage behavior. A combination of medication and counseling—and monitoring the condition for a lifetime—forms the most common treatment plan.

If a child in your life is chronically angry and irritable and prone to sudden temper outbursts, he or she may be suffering from disruptive mood dysregulation disorder, or DMDD—a condition named only recently, in 2013. With some symptoms similar to attention deficit disorder, it may be treated with similar counseling and medication. (See Attention-Deficit/Hyperactivity Disorders, page 76.) While several drugs are currently in testing, the NIH recommends psychotherapy as the first approach, with medications added depending on the symptoms. CBD may have a future with all these conditions.

WHAT CBD CAN DO: In both schizophrenia and bipolar disorder, it appears that people have physical changes in the structure of their brain and nervous system. In schizophrenia, scientists believe that the ECS plays a role in releasing certain brain chemicals that may contribute to symptoms. While CBD's inherent anti-inflammatory and neuroprotective qualities have been seen to aid brain health in general, CBD may also play a part in the ECS release of the endocannabinoid anandamide, which in the right amounts appears to act like an antipsychotic drug. A study on schizophrenic patients published in a 2018 issue of *American Journal of Psychiatry* used CBD to supplement regular antipsychotic medication and found that CBD users improved significantly compared to a placebo group. Several other studies support CBD's positive action: 2015 research in *Neurotherapeutics* touts CBD's "therapeutic potential" for treating schizophrenia, saying it likely has "better tolerability than antipsychotic treatments," and a 2012 study at Germany's University of Cologne found that both CBD and a mainstream antipsychotic drug had an equal measure of improvement—while CBD had no side effects. Scientists are unsure how bipolar disorder is linked to the ECS, and studies are ongoing. But CBD does have an impact on the depression that accompanies the "low" and the anxiety that can come with the "high." (See Depression, page 69, and Anxiety, page 67.) Experts recommend CBD dosing based on treating those symptoms. Deanna Gabriel Vierck, who works with families whose children have ADHD or symptoms of DMDD, with anger outbursts and general impatience, has found that CBD is widely used by them (see Attention-Deficit/Hyperactivity Disorders, page 76).

NOTE: It's important to know that while many have self-medicated with CBD's cannabinoid cousin THC for both schizophrenia and bipolar disorder, THC's effect is often opposite that of soothing CBD, and it can make symptoms worse, increasing anxiety, paranoia, and other undesirable feelings.

DELIVERY METHODS

* Ingested: capsule, sublingual tincture, concentrate, spray or drop, nano/liposomal oil, and edible for long-term anti-inflammatory and neuroprotection benefits, calming benefits, anxiety relief, and possible antipsychotic effects (usually for CBD-THC strains; still being studied).

* Inhaled: vaporizing pen for anxiety relief, mood lift.

Skin Conditions: Eczema, Hives, Psoriasis, Dandruff, Acne

The skin is your largest organ. Daily it protects your entire body, rids it of toxins, and blocks invading microorganisms. That doesn't mean you should hibernate. Skin also needs the right amount of sun-sent vitamin D to regenerate cells and to build strong bones and inner organs; and exercise in the fresh air improves circulation, which keeps skin functioning at top levels—and makes it glow without makeup. Keeping your skin healthy is also dependent on regenerative sleep; stress management; eating cleansing, antioxidant fruits and vegetables; and drinking plenty of water. Even with all this, environmental factors can sometimes trigger inflammation, a condition called dermatitis (*derma* means "skin").

Poison ivy or oak, topical antibiotics, and detergents are all instigators. Radiation for cancer patients can cause it, too. In other cases, allergies are responsible. Red, itchy, scaly patches, which sometimes become crusty and ooze, may signal eczema. Hives are another allergic reaction in which small, red, itchy bumps appear. The source of the reaction may be hard to identify—but once you do find it, be sure to stay away. Exposure can make it worse each time. Psoriasis is an autoimmune disease; that is, the immune system triggers it, causing inflammation on the skin and inside the body. Normally as new skin forms, old skin sloughs off. In this case, the old cells remain. The pileup causes raised red patches called plaques— usually appearing on the scalp, elbows, buttocks, and knees. A few triggers may be infection, tobacco smoke, and gluten in the diet. Both psoriasis and eczema, like other skin infections, can cause the scalp to flake, bringing undesirable dandruff.

And there is acne, the bane of a teenager's existence (but adults can develop it, too). Basically, hair follicles fill with oil from sebaceous (oil) glands below them, bacteria finds its way in, and the follicle becomes infected. The face, shoulders, chest, and back, the areas most populated by sebaceous glands, are prime acne sites. Hormones, medications, stress, and diet all may play a part in triggering acne.

In all cases, practice skin health: shower quickly in warm, not hot, water (hot water dries it out); don't smoke, since smoking depletes oxygen and nutrients; moisturize daily with SPF to guard against dangerous ultraviolet rays; get plenty of sleep; and eat well. CBD is developing rave reviews for skin support, too.

WHAT CBD CAN DO: Because skin has the highest number and concentration of CB2 receptors in the body, the ECS obviously plays a major part in skin health. Research shows that cannabinoids like CBD can interact with the CB2 receptors to calm inflammation. A 2006 study in Germany showed that cannabinoid-rich products applied to sites with eczema and other skin inflammations soothed itching. In the case of psoriasis, CBD and other cannabinoids appear to inhibit the overproliferation of cells that cause the pileup of skin cells and plaque. Hemp seed oil has also been used on eczema with success. A 2018 report in the *International Journal of Molecular Sciences* backed up the lubricating and healing benefits of plant oils for keeping the skin barrier strong against environmental invaders, and for being antioxidant, anti-inflammatory, and antimicrobial; wound healing; and anticarcinogenic. For acne treatment, CBD has been found to specifically deliver antiacne activity by tamping down oil production from sebaceous glands and lowering inflammation. The supporting cast in the cannabis plant includes the terpenes limonene, which fights bacteria involved in acne infection, and linalool, which works against inflammation.

DELIVERY SYSTEMS

* Ingested: capsule, sublingual tincture, concentrate, spray or drop, nano/ liposomal oil, isolates, edibles to fight internal triggers for inflammation, cell and gland overproduction, and infection, depending on the condition. Hemp seed oil with plentiful omega-3s may help to control inflammation.

* Topical: salves, balms, lotions, oils for inflammation, itching, and infection, depending on condition; especially helpful when used in combination with ingested CBD.

Stroke and Traumatic Brain Injury

According to the Centers for Disease Control, some 75 million Americans suffer from high blood pressure, or hypertension, which leads to the two top killers in the nation: heart disease and stroke. As we age, arteries lose flexibility and fatty deposits collect on artery walls, gradually making them stiff and narrow and reducing healthy blood flow. This causes hypertension, or high blood pressure, as the heart works harder to move blood through arteries. Eventually fatty buildup may block blood flow to the brain or a weakened artery may burst. A stroke happens. Sudden numbness or weakness on one side of the body; severe headache; confusion; or trouble speaking, seeing, and walking are all signs. If you notice these symptoms, call 911 immediately. According to the National Stroke Association, nearly one million people each year suffer stroke—about one every 40 seconds. The good news is that 80 percent of strokes be prevented. While a tendency toward stroke can be hereditary, strokes can also be triggered by atrial fibrillation (irregular heartbeat), by certain medications, or by preventable triggers: smoking, a diet high in fat and sugar, lack of exercise or sleep, and continual stress. No one is bulletproof: stroke can happen at any age. To help stop stroke in its tracks, make some lifestyle changes. Start with exercise, which lowers blood pressure and bad cholesterol, and a Mediterranean diet, which means one rich in fruits, vegetables, and healthy fats that come from extra-virgin olive oil and nuts. A 2018 issue of the *New England Journal of Medicine* reports on a Spanish study in which participants showed lower incidence of heart disease and stroke after following a Mediterranean diet for five years.

While stroke is an inner injury, other traumatic brain injuries (TBIs) are triggered by outside events. Few people are strangers to a head bump and the localized swelling, or "egg," that pops up. This means that a blood vessel tore under the scalp, and with the application of cold packs, it will gradually subside. Other internal head injuries are more serious. Chronic traumatic encephalopathy occurs after a series of concussions—events in which the head is shaken or struck so that the brain bangs against the skull, becoming bruised. A concussion from a sports impact, a car accident, or a fall or other blunt force can knock a person out and cause brain bleeding, swelling, severe headache, and long-term neurological damage. For some, bed rest and care can bring things back to normal. For others, permanent body and brain damage require long-term therapy. After many concussions, CTE may develop. The term strikes fear in the hearts of football players and other professional athletes: over time, memory loss, confusion, aggression, Parkinson's, and dementia have led many to suicide. Avoiding sports that revolve around serious impact with each move is one way to avoid CTE. Otherwise, take extreme care as you drive, walk stairs, and, generally, live. CBD is showing potentially beneficial uses.

WHAT CBD CAN DO: Because the ECS and its receptors CB1 and CB2 regulate key brain function such as blood flow, inflammation, and plasticity, CBD and THC can play a key role in supporting the ECS to keep the brain strong and help it make a comeback from injury. Both are antioxidant and neuroprotectant: They help keep brain cells healthy to better fight a medical insult. One theory is that when an internal stroke or external impact injury occurs, the CB1 receptors concentrated in the brain react by sending out inflammatory compounds in addition to cell-damaging free radicals. Brain tissue swells, veins deteriorate, and cells die. CBD and other cannabinoids can race to the rescue: As well as being naturally anti-inflammatory and antioxidant, they likely interact with CB1 receptors to help arrest brain swelling and counteract cell death. Recent animal studies show that, in addition, CBD regulates heart arrhythmia, or irregular heartbeat, which can cause stroke. To fight traumatic brain injury, CB2 receptors, which populate the immune, metabolic, and peripheral nervous systems, have been found to increase in number during and immediately after a TBI. They likely help modulate inflammation and vein damage, says research in a 2014 issue of *Journal of Neuroinflammation*. Research also shows that CBD and THC likely boost the activity of these receptors, to help support their mission. Members of the National Football League have been promoting research on CBD and THC to help address injury from concussion and the pain that accompanies it. A 2017 article in *Frontiers of Pharmacology* supports CBD's potential use to ease neurological side effects, including spinal cord injury, that players suffer after brain impact. Since 2017, an initiative called When the Bright Lights Fade is working with former NFL players and scientists from Maryland's Johns Hopkins University and the University of Pennsylvania to study CBD's "capacity to relieve pain from injury and counteract the disturbing symptoms of CTE." Outside this project, the internet is filled with testimonials from football, hockey, martial arts, and other athletes who have found relief.

DELIVERY METHODS

* Ingested: capsule, sublingual tincture, concentrate, spray or drop, nano/liposomal oil, edibles for pain and for long-term anti-inflammatory, antioxidant, and neuroprotection benefits.

* Inhaled: vaporizing pen for acute anxiety, pain.

Women's Health

Every woman in the world is destined for two major changes in life: menstruation and menopause. While each signals important and beautiful milestones in life, each is also accompanied by symptoms that don't make life easy, to say the least. For more than 90 percent of women, menstruation is accompanied by premenstrual syndrome, reports the Health and Human Services Office on Women's Health. That means just before their period, they'll experience one or several symptoms that doctors think are related to fluctuation of hormones at this time of month: abdominal bloating, cramping, headaches, breast tenderness, moodiness, carbohydrate cravings, anxiety, and depression—sometimes so debilitating that the only way to deal is to lie in bed with a hot water bottle while work, school, and the world pass by. Once menstrual flow begins, the pain largely disappears (cramping may remain), only to return in a few weeks. The unpleasant monthly buildup seems to peak in a woman's 30s and then gradually dissipate. Menopause signals the end of menstruation, the loss of fertility, and a move toward the twilight years. But don't think it's an easy slide into home plate. Hot flashes and night sweats announce the change, sometimes with perspiration so severe that it necessitates a change of clothes during the day or sheets in the wee hours. Vaginal dryness, insomnia, slowing metabolism with weight gain, and thinning nails and hair can visit a person during this time. Bone loss quickens, and osteoporosis can set in (see Bone Health and Osteoporosis, page 81). If menstrual pain is especially severe, it may indicate disease, such as endometriosis. This develops when the endometrium, or tissue that lines the inside of the uterus, migrates to the outside. It irritates other tissue and causes scar tissue to form around the uterus, ovaries, and fallopian tubes. Severe pelvic pain and excessive bleeding can happen during menstruation, along with pain during intercourse and/or urination. It may inhibit fertility and be a step toward ovarian cancer. For PMS, help can come in the form of aspirin, ibuprofen, or heat application. Sometimes a doctor will prescribe hormonal medication, such as birth control pills, to balance the fluctuation of estrogen and progesterone; antidepressants and antianxiety medicine for emotional swings; or diuretics for bloating. To alleviate menopause discomfort, a doctor may prescribe small amounts of estrogen. If it's exceptionally painful and inhibiting fertility, endometriosis may require surgery.

No one feels like moving when suffering pain, but believe it or not, exercise can help with menstrual cramps. Eating a diet rich in anti-inflammatory fruits and vegetables—and not giving in to carb and sugar cravings—will help control bloating and mood swings. CBD is finding its way into the list of remedies.

WHAT CBD CAN DO: In women, receptors appear to have high concentration in the uterus and other parts of the reproductive system, and a study in the 2016 *Reproduction* journal reports that endocannabinoids likely interact with those receptors to play a role in fertility and egg implantation. Research shows that CBD and other cannabinoids may play a role in supporting fertility. Scientists agree that there is much work still to do to determine the role of the ECS and cannabinoids in women's health. But they do know that both play a role in easing a woman's anxiety and stress, to aid in conception. (See Anxiety, page 67, and Stress, 63.) For the cramps and bloating that accompany PMS, CBD has been shown to ease pain and inflammation (see Pain, page 112, and Inflammation, pages 62–63). Aside from CBD, the omega-3 and omega-6 fatty acids in hemp seed oil have been found to help stabilize the fluctuating blood sugar levels that may contribute to PMS. In the case of menopause, the ECS appears to have lost tone and to be endocannabinoid deficient. Cannabinoids may help return balance. Cannabis in the form of THC has been reported to ease hot flashes, and CBD has been found helpful in alleviating the depression and bone loss that can accompany this change in life (see Depression, page 69, and Bone Health, pages 81–82). For endometriosis, research shows that CBD, often combined with THC, helps to ameliorate endometriosis by inhibiting tissue from migrating outside the uterus.

DELIVERY SYSTEMS

* Ingested: capsule, sublingual tincture, concentrate, spray or drop, nano/ liposomal oil, edibles, isolates to ease anxiety and lift mood, relieve pain from cramps, lessen inflammation that causes bloating in PMS, inhibit bone loss in menopause, and halt endometriosis spread. Hemp seed oil high in omega-3s may help stabilize high-sugar food cravings.

* Inhaled: vaporizing pen for acute anxiety, stress, and pain.

* Topical: salves, balms, lotions, oils for abdominal massage for PMS, menstrual, and endometrial pain.

Wounds: Cuts, Bruises, Burns

A scrape while sliding into home plate; a cut while pulling a knife out of the dishwasher; a bruise after surgery or from banging into furniture in the middle of the night; a hot-pan burn while cooking. These are frustrating and inconvenient, and they hurt. In the case of small wounds, we set a stiff upper lip and carry on. Knowing how to treat them quickly keeps wounds from growing into more severe problems. With a cut or scrape, let it bleed a little, which actually helps clean it. Then wash it in two rounds, with cool to warm running water and mild soap (not antibacterial, which may contain triclosan, which may promote resistance to healing). Remove bits of gravel, glass, grass, etc., that may have wedged in under the skin. Then cover it with a sterile bandage, changing it daily or when wet. For deeper cuts, place a clean cloth or piece of gauze over it and apply pressure for at least five minutes to help the blood clot. If it soaks through, add more cloth or gauze on top of the existing one—and don't lift to look, which interrupts the clotting. For a puncture wound, after cleaning it thoroughly, keep it uncovered so that it heals from the inside out; if the skin heals first, it may trap bacteria inside. A bruise is a horse of a different color, literally. A bang or bump can break blood vessels in tissue, causing it to swell as a beautiful eggplant-colored burst of blood spreads out beneath the skin. The injured tissue is tender. As it heals, the spilled blood cells break down, turning the area green and yellow before it returns to its normal color and size. Cold compresses or an ice pack immediately help arrest swelling, and the anti-inflammatory herbs touted for centuries—like Saint John's wort, aloe, and arnica massaged into the skin—work for days afterward to stop the spread of subdural bleeding and help the blood aura to dissipate. A burn can happen in the kitchen, under the hot sun, or while working with chemicals. A first-degree burn causes redness and possibly peeling on the top layer of skin; a second-degree burn goes a layer deeper and triggers blistering; a third-degree burn is serious, involving damaged to tissue and possibly nerves. Varied levels of pain accompany each. In the case of the first two, quickly plunging the area into cool water for three to five minutes can help stop the burning; then wash with mild soap and water, and cover with gauze to keep out bacteria. Aloe, honey, and green tea are anti-inflammatory and antibacterial and can help speed healing for the first two burns—so can CBD products. For third-degree burns, call 911.

WHAT CBD CAN DO: Little did ancient healers know that their success in treating wounds with cannabis would hold up for thousands of years. An article in the 2017 *Journal of Pain Symptom Management* notes that "topical medical cannabis has the potential to improve pain management in patients suffering from wounds of all classes. Today, many experts link healing by cannabinoid to the ECS. Research shows that CB1 and CB2 receptors spring up at wound sites, possibly encouraging the inflammation and other reactions involved in healing for cuts, burns, and bruises. CBD may interact with these receptors to continue the healing process. Its inherent antibacterial, anti-inflammatory, and analgesic, or pain-relieving, powers make it a soothing, healing medicine when applied to the skin or taken internally. (See Antibiotic-Resistant Bacterial Infection, page 72, and Chronic Pain, page 112.) In addition, it works with receptors to grow new skin over wounds and burns. For bruises, CBD added to other anti-inflammatory and antioxidant plant oils such as olive and jojoba, and massaged into the injured area helps break up blood clotting beneath the skin and soothe the pain of impact that caused the bruise. Sometimes the healing process goes awry and blood clots can form, embedding in the lungs, heart, or brain and causing life-threatening events. Natural blood thinners, omega-3s are found in CBD's cousin hemp oil and have been found to help prevent clots from forming and new ones from growing.

DELIVERY METHODS

* Ingested: capsule, sublingual tincture, concentrate, spray or drop, nano/liposomal oil, edibles for antioxidant, anti-inflammatory, pain-relieving, and anti-itching benefits.

* Inhaled: vaporizing pen for acute pain.

* Topical: salves, balms, lotions, oils for antibacterial, anti-inflammatory, pain-relieving, and skin-binding effects.

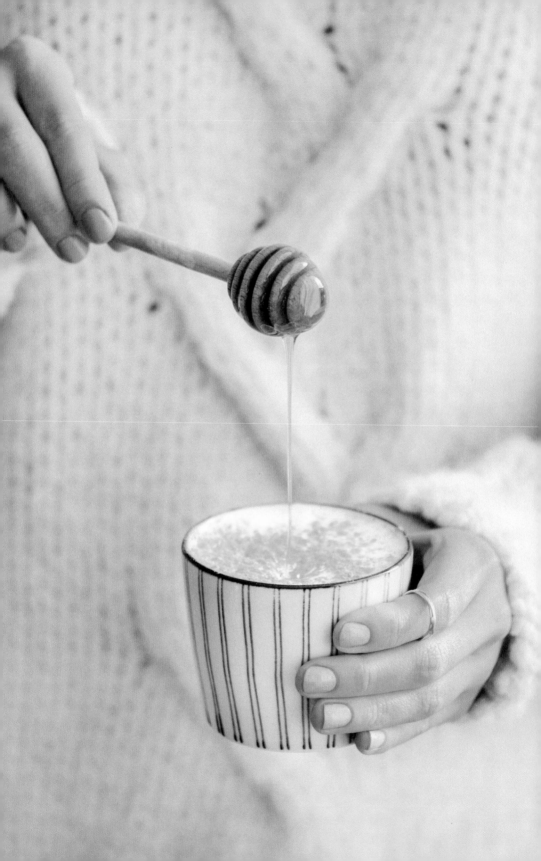

PART FOUR

RECIPES

Now that you know all about CBD and what you want it to do for you, it's time to put your CBD product to work! We hope you'll try and enjoy the CBD-rich recipes below. They're divided into five categories: *Beverages, Little Bites, Big Bites, Topicals,* and *Tinctures and Tonics.* For each, you'll discover what other nutritional value they bring to help you manage a condition or boost your overall wellness. Put on your chef's hat and get into the kitchen—you'll like the results!

Dosage Guidelines

Before you start, work with your CBD-savvy health care professional to find a product you like and to determine how much you'll need. At the end of the day, you have to explore what's right for your body, and the dosage depends on:

1. Your condition and its intensity
2. Your body weight, composition, and metabolism
3. Your endocannabinoid system's "tone" and ability to adjust to gradual use of CBD
4. Your general reaction to any cannabis product

For the recipes below, we recommend using this rule of thumb:

* One dose of CBD supplement = between 4 milligrams and 30 milligrams for each serving. You may find you'll want a slightly lower or higher dosage. As always, begin low and titrate, or work up gradually.

* For each serving of food or drink or ingested medicinal, we recommend using 1 dose of CBD supplement, depending on what you determine your dose to be.

* For the topical medicinals such as salves or massage oils, we've given you specific measures of CBD for each recipe. That's because uptake is not quite as fast as with ingested foods, and there is less need to carefully titrate.

* Follow the dosage guidelines on page 54 to determine how many drops or teaspoons of CBD make up a dose based on the concentration of CBD per bottle. Some bottles hold 250 mg of CBD per ounce; others hold 50 mg CBD per ounce; and still others hold 1,000 mg CBD per ounce.

Here are some examples using the lowest recommended dosage of 4 milligrams CBD per serving for the recipes below:

CBD Milky Turmeric Tea (page 136)
Recipe makes: 2 (1-cup) servings
1 dose of CBD oil per serving: 4 mg
Doses of CBD for entire recipe: 2 doses or 8 mg

Elderberry Syrup (page 202)
16 (1-tablespoon) servings
4 mg CBD oil per serving
16 doses or 64 mg in recipe

Nerve Tonic Tincture (page 204)
22 (½-teaspoon or 2-drop) servings (in a 1-ounce bottle of 44 dropperfuls)
4 mg CBD oil per serving
22 doses or 88 mg in recipe

CBD Product Guidelines

Look back to Know Delivery Systems in Part One (page 37) for the supplements you'd like to use for the following recipes. We recommend choosing among these three:

* Tinctures (alcohol-based or oil-based) and glycerites
* Isolate powders
* Nano-liposomal oils

Whenever possible below, we'll offer specific suggestions on the forms to use. If there are multiple good options for the recipe, we'll suggest doses of "CBD supplement" and you can choose the form you like.

Remember: Heat changes cannabinoids. So always add your CBD at the end of creating a heated product.

Your CBD Kitchen

In the following pages, you'll discover 43 recipes with nutrient-rich ingredients enhanced by hemp CBD supplements. Because you're not extracting your own hemp CBD oil from the fresh hemp plant, but rather adding the manufactured CBD product to food and drink recipes, your kitchen will be less like a CBD apothecary and more like an organic chef's kitchen, filled with herbs, spices, fruits, vegetables, and oils. Here are a few utensils you'll need to whip up these soothing delights:

* Baking pans
* Blender or food processor
* Double boiler
* Glass pint and quart jars with lids
* Measuring cup
* Mixing bowls

* Mixing spoons and spatulas
* Molds (for gummies, pops, and bath bombs)
* Plastic storage containers
* Pitcher
* Whisk

Have fun!

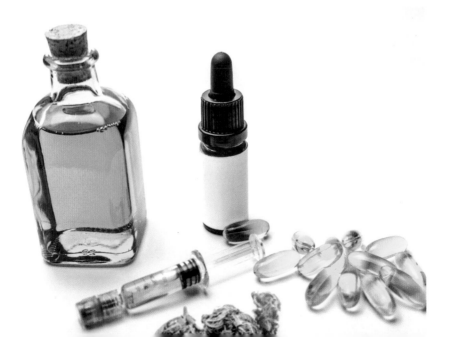

CBD MILKY TURMERIC TEA
Compliments of Lynn Brownell and Katie Brownell

My sister-in-law Lynn and my niece Katie, who is an organic farmer, share this divinely soothing and inflammation-fighting tea. Turmeric contains curcumin, which is anti-inflammatory, antioxidant, and antimicrobial. Ginger is a longtime natural antidote for rheumatoid arthritis.

2 (1-cup) servings

WHAT YOU'LL NEED:

½ cup water

1 teaspoon turmeric powder

1-inch piece ginger, peeled and grated

2 pods cardamom

2 cinnamon sticks

6 black peppercorns

1 tablespoon honey

2 bags or 1 tablespoon loose leaf black chai or green tea

2 cups almond milk

2 doses CBD oil-based supplement, either oil-based tincture or nano-liposomal oil

WHAT YOU'LL DO:

1. In a small saucepan over low heat, add the water, turmeric, ginger, cardamom, cinnamon, peppercorns, honey, and tea. Bring to a simmer, then pour in milk and stir.

2. When milk is steaming, use a spoon to taste; add more honey as needed.

3. Pour into 2 cups through a fine-mesh strainer to remove the loose tea leaves.

4. Add a dose of CBD oil to each cup and drink while hot.

* Inflammation (including arthritis, asthma, stroke, neurodegenerative disease)

* Insomnia

* Bone health

* Immune system enhancement

BACTERIA-FIGHTING SMOOTHIE

Cranberries are known universally for their UTI-fighting abilities, but studies show that the juice alone doesn't have enough active ingredients to inhibit bacteria from attacking the bladder wall. The probiotics in kefir boost urinary tract health, as does the fiber in oats. Deanna suggests using an orange-flavored CBD oil-based supplement for an added citrus flavor.

2 servings

WHAT YOU'LL NEED:

1 cup unsweetened cranberry juice

2 cups whole cranberries

1 frozen banana

½ cup plain kefir

1 tablespoon hemp seeds

3 tablespoons rolled oats

2 tablespoons honey

2 doses CBD oil-based supplement, either oil-based tincture or nano-liposomal oil

WHAT YOU'LL DO:

1. Place all ingredients in a blender and blend until smooth. Taste, and add another tablespoon of honey if too tart. If so, blend to incorporate the honey and serve.

ALTERNATIVE: This recipe can be made with 1 cup apple or orange juice for a different punch.

WHAT YOU'LL USE IT FOR:

* Bladder health

* Asthma

* Diabetes

* Digestive disorders

* Heart health

* Liver disease

* Prostate health

* Metabolic syndrome

CBD MOCK-POLITAN

Put your feet up with this non-alcoholic cocktail combining the antioxidant and anti-inflammatory benefits of cranberry and lime. According to the Mayo Clinic, the scent of citrus is a valuable stress reliever. Plus, CBD's calming benefits will leave you relaxed.

1 serving

WHAT YOU'LL NEED:

⅔ cup cranberry juice

⅓ cup lemon or lime-flavored sparkling water

2 tablespoons cranberry-orange CBD syrup (page 139)

1 tablespoon freshly squeezed lime juice

Ice cubes

Orange twist and fresh frozen cranberries, for garnish

WHAT YOU'LL DO:

1. In a cocktail shaker, combine the cranberry juice, cranberry-orange CBD syrup, lime juice, and ice, and shake thoroughly.

2. Strain into a chilled martini glass and garnish with orange twist and fresh frozen cranberries before serving.

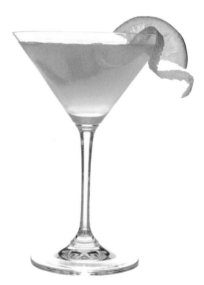

CRANBERRY-ORANGE CBD SYRUP
Compliments of Deanna Gabriel Vierck

10 (2-tablespoon) servings

WHAT YOU'LL NEED:

1 (8 ounce) bag organic cranberries

1 whole organic orange, sliced and chopped into smaller pieces

1½ cups water

¼ cup honey

10 doses CBD isolate or oil-based supplement, either oil-based tincture or nano-liposomal oil

WHAT YOU'LL DO:

1. Place the cranberries, orange, and water in a small saucepan and cook over medium-low heat for 20 minutes, stirring occasionally.

2. Turn off heat and allow ingredients to cool for 20 minutes, stirring occasionally.

3. Strain through a fine-mesh metal strainer. You should have approximately 1 cup of liquid.

4. Add honey while still warm and mix to combine thoroughly. Allow the liquid to cool.

5. Once completely cooled, add the CBD. Store in a glass bottle in refrigerator for up to 2 months.

WHAT YOU'LL USE IT FOR:

* Stress

* Anxiety

* Inflammation

* Bladder health

* Heart health

* Cancer protection

* Liver disease

* Immune system enhancement

LAVENDER-GINGER CORDIAL

Deanna says: "Lavender and ginger can work together as an internal remedy for a headache, but treating a headache depends on the quality—full or deficient. When the head feels full, lavender is great for draining and calming. If it hurts to touch the head, ginger could be more helpful as it encourages more blood flow. Both are anti-inflammatory and antispasmodic, helping ease tension headache. Plus, ginger keeps nausea in check."

2 servings

WHAT YOU'LL NEED:

3 cups water

½ cup grated ginger root

4 cardamom pods, opened

½ stick cinnamon

5 cloves

1 star fruit, sliced

1 lemon, peeled and juiced

10 drops lavender essential oil

1 tablespoon honey

2 doses CBD isolate or oil-based supplement, either oil-based tincture or nano-liposomal oil

WHAT YOU'LL DO:

1. In a pan over medium-high heat, bring the water, all the spices, and the star fruit slices to a boil. Then cover and simmer for 20 minutes.

2. Remove from the burner and add the lemon juice and peel; allow to steep for 2–3 hours.

3. Pour the liquid through a strainer into a glass pint jar. Stir in the lavender essential oil, honey, and CBD, and cap tightly. Refrigerate for 3–5 days.

4. When you feel a headache coming on, sip ¼ cup, or stir ¼ cup with ¼ cup of either hot water, apple, or cranberry juice. Close your eyes and relax as you sip.

NOTE: Deanna says: "Be sure to decrease the ginger if the head feels full— you'll want the effect of the lavender. Decrease the lavender if the head feels deficient—you'll want more ginger to increase blood flow."

WHAT YOU'LL USE IT FOR:

* Headache
* Inflammation
* Digestive health
* Heart health
* Nausea and vomiting

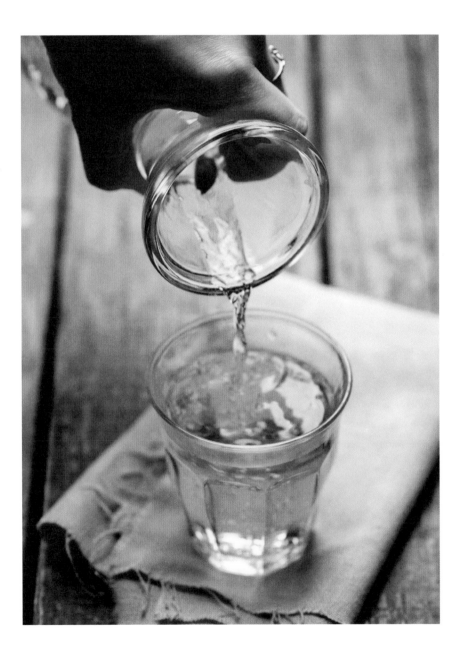

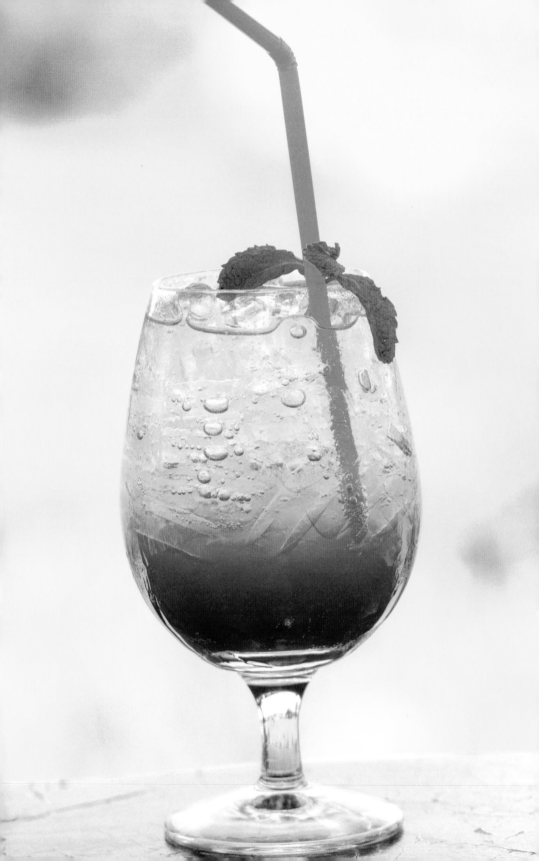

PRICKLY PEAR MOCKTAIL

Thanks to a study in 2004, prickly pear juice has been touted as a hangover remedy; it was shown to aid recovery time and protect liver cells from alcohol damage. Enjoy this tasty drink full of antioxidants and anti-inflammatory benefits with a steamed artichoke—a member of the liver-nutritious milk thistle family—dipped in melted ghee or clarified butter (page 154).

1 serving

WHAT YOU'LL NEED:

2 large or 3 small prickly pears, preferably with spines removed; if not, see step 1 for removal tips

1 teaspoon lime juice

1 teaspoon honey

1 dose CBD isolate or oil-based supplement, either oil-based tincture or nano-liposomal oil

Mint leaves, for garnish

Sparkling water

WHAT YOU'LL DO:

1. If the prickly pear spines are intact, remove them by blanching and dissolving them in a pan of boiling water (while wearing rubber gloves!).

2. Cut the pears in half and scoop out the flesh. Place in a blender and puree until smooth.

3. Strain the pureed fruit through a sieve and into a large measuring cup to remove any remaining seeds. You will have about ⅓ cup prickly pear juice.

4. Pour the juice into a cocktail shaker, and add the lime juice, honey, and CBD. Shake until well blended.

5. Pour juice over ice cubes into an 8- or 12-ounce glass. Add a mint garnish.

6. Add desired amount of sparkling water for an extra zing.

ALTERNATIVE: Place a twist of lime rind in each ice cube before freezing for an added garnish before serving.

WHAT YOU'LL USE IT FOR:

* Liver health

* Inflammation

* Heart health

AVOCADO SMOOTHIE

Foods rich in omega-3s fight inflammation in the brain and body and help relieve a range of ailments, from depression and brain injury to digestive and heart conditions. Avocado and hemp seeds top the list. Ginger and turmeric are also neuroinflammation fighters; some experts recommend 1 teaspoon of turmeric a day to keep inflammation in check. Fruits and vegetables carry antioxidant (cell-protecting) flavonols. Doctors at the Mayo Clinic also recommend supplementing any diet with bone-supporting vitamin D, which includes milk, coconut milk, and some yogurts (be sure they are D-fortified).

2–3 servings

WHAT YOU'LL NEED:

1 ripe avocado, sliced and frozen

1 large handful of kale or spinach

1 banana, frozen

½ cup unsweetened coconut milk

½ cup plain vitamin D-fortified yogurt

1 tablespoon honey

1 teaspoon fresh grated ginger

½ teaspoon turmeric powder

1 tablespoon hemp seeds

2 doses CBD isolate or oil-based supplement, either oil-based tincture or nano-liposomal oil

WHAT YOU'LL DO:

1. In a blender, add the avocado, kale, banana, coconut milk, yogurt, and honey and blend to combine. Add the ginger, turmeric, hemp seeds, and CBD oil. Blend until smooth and serve.

WHAT YOU'LL USE IT FOR:

* Multiple sclerosis

* Inflammation

* Bone health

* Depression

* Digestive health

* Heart health

* Neurodegenerative disease

* Psychological health

* Stroke and traumatic brain injury

FRESH GINGER TEA

Ginger tea is a time-honored nausea queller that calms the lining of the stomach. Try to use fresh instead of powdered ginger or ginger tea bags—the freshest nutrients act most quickly. Lemon and orange boost essential vitamin C, and if you're battling flu, try an added pinch of antibacterial cayenne.

2 servings

WHAT YOU'LL NEED:

2 cups water

Six ¼-inch slices ginger root, peeled and diced

2 teaspoons honey

Juice of 2 lemon quarters and

2 orange quarters

Pinch of cayenne (optional)

2 doses CBD isolate or oil-based supplement, either oil-based tincture or nano-liposomal oil

WHAT YOU'LL DO:

1. In a pan, boil the water. Once boiling, add the ginger root and simmer for 10 minutes.

2. Cover the pan and remove it from the heat, allowing the ginger to steep for 15 additional minutes.

3. Strain out the ginger root and pour it into two cups.

4. Into each cup, stir 1 teaspoon of honey and the juice of 1 lemon slice and 1 orange slice. Add a pinch of cayenne if you'd like.

5. Stir in CBD and serve.

ALTERNATIVE: Deanna says: "Make a ginger spritzer. Use the same ingredients, but reduce the water to ½ cup, divide the strained tea into two ¼-cup servings, and add the honey and lemon, orange, and cayenne if you like. Then add unflavored club soda to each serving. The carbonation and addition of minerals like sodium bicarbonate in club soda can also be helpful for nausea."

NOTE: If you need immediate action, pour 1 cup of boiled water over ½ teaspoon powdered ginger, steep for as long as you can, and then strain out the ginger through a coffee filter. Or use a ginger tea bag.

WHAT YOU'LL USE IT FOR:

* Nausea and vomiting
* Chemotherapy
* Headache
* Heart health

* Inflammation
* Women's health (menopause and PMS)

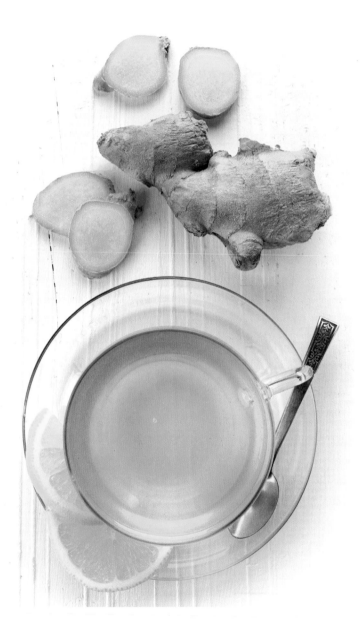

LEMONADE
Compliments of Deanna Gabriel Vierck

Deanna says: "This drink is a favorite in my house, and my 5-year-old son often requests it! While it's a good-tasting, low-sugar drink in general, it's fantastic for those recovering from colds and flu. Lemon juice is often praised for its benefits for liver and digestive health, and its trace minerals are wonderful for maintaining and supporting health. The sodium ascorbate is a form of vitamin C for stubborn chest congestion, and there is much research on the benefits of vitamin D for preventing illness and recovering from an acute bout."

1 serving

WHAT YOU'LL NEED:

2½ tablespoons lemon juice

¼–½ teaspoons sodium ascorbate (vitamin C) powder

⅛ teaspoon sea salt

1½–2 teaspoons maple syrup

1 dose of liquid vitamin D, available in drops and sprays

1 cup water

1 dose CBD isolate or oil-based supplement, either oil-based tincture or nano-liposomal oil

WHAT YOU'LL DO:

1. Place all ingredients in a glass and stir gently until combined well.

ALTERNATIVE: Add a teaspoon of elderberry syrup (page 202) for an additional immune boost.

NOTE: Follow the dosage directions on the bottle of liquid vitamin D.

WHAT YOU'LL USE IT FOR:

* Inflammation (from colds and flu)

* Asthma

* Immune System enhancement (cellular function and lymphatic health

* Pain (including exercise recovery)

* Headache from dehydration

* Nausea and Vomiting (recovery from dehydration)

* Bone health (and related muscle health)

SWEET HEMP MILK
Compliments of Deanna Gabriel Vierck and Julia Kay

Deanna says: "My good friend Julia Kay created a similar recipe to help make her CBD supplement more palatable for her young daughter who was struggling with toddler tantrums and mood swings. It worked like a charm! And hemp milk is rich in anti-inflammatory omega-3s, and good for heart and brain health. This is a great recipe for anyone who doesn't prefer the taste of CBD and needs a quick, simple way to ingest it."

1 serving

WHAT YOU'LL NEED:

¾ cup or 6 ounces unsweetened hemp, almond, or coconut milk

2 teaspoons maple syrup or honey

1 dose CBD isolate or oil-based supplement, either oil-based tincture or nano-liposomal oil

WHAT YOU'LL DO:

1. Mix all ingredients in a glass, stir well, and drink immediately. If using honey, you will need to stir longer for it to dissolve.

ALTERNATIVE: Deanna says: "Replace the milks above with this easy elderberry milk. Add 1 tablespoon of the elderberry syrup (page 202) to ¾ cup of the unsweetened milk of your choice."

WHAT YOU'LL USE IT FOR:

* ADHD

* Stress

* Anxiety

* Insomnia

* Heart health

* Bone health

* Neurodegenerative conditions

REISHI GOLDEN MILK
Compliments of Deanna Gabriel Vierck

Deanna says: "Reishi mushrooms are incredible for immune function. The most medicinal form is tea, but the taste can be a challenge. I often make this golden milk—a coconut milk reishi chai that's spice-forward and thus pretty tasty."

6 servings

WHAT YOU'LL NEED:

- 1 whole reishi mushroom about 6–8 inches wide or about 13 reishi mushroom slices
- One 2-inch piece of fresh ginger, chopped, or 1 tablespoon of dried ginger root, adjusting more or less depending on how spicy you like your chai
- 2 teaspoons cinnamon chips or 2 cinnamon sticks
- 2 teaspoons black peppercorns
- 1 teaspoon clove powder or 8–10 whole cloves
- 1 teaspoon cardamom hulls
- 2 teaspoon licorice root (this will sweeten the tea and eliminate the need to add additional sugar)
- 6 cups water
- ½ can full-fat coconut milk
- 6 doses CBD isolate or oil-based supplement, either oil-based tincture or nano-liposomal oil

WHAT YOU'LL DO:

1. Place all herbs and spices in a large stockpot and cover with water.

2. Bring to a gentle simmer and continue for at least 1 hour before serving. This will allow more of the reishi compounds to release and offer a rich and complex flavor.

3. After cooking tea for about an hour, add coconut milk. It is fine to allow the tea to continue to simmer after adding the coconut milk.

4. Pour or ladle tea through a fine mesh strainer to remove the herb pieces.

5. Add a dose of CBD to each individual cup. Sip slowly and allow the tea to linger in your mouth to increase absorption of desired herbal compounds.

ALTERNATIVE: Deanna says: "I often leave my pot of tea simmering all day and just strain single cups while leaving the rest in the pot to continue simmering. The effects on the flavor and medicinal benefit are wonderful!"

WHAT YOU'LL USE IT FOR:

* Immune system enhancement
* Fibromyalgia
* Insomnia
* Inflammation
* Pain and chronic pain
* Stress

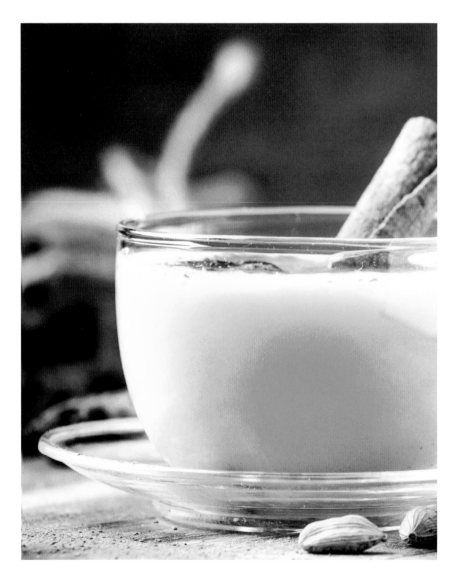

CBD SLEEPYTIME GUMMIES

Combined with CBD and soothing antioxidant and anti-inflammatory green tea, these gummies pave a new way to sleep. An anti-inflammatory, tart cherry juice has pain-relieving properties, too, especially for muscle, joint, and nerve pain.

10–12 servings

WHAT YOU'LL NEED:

1 cup tart cherry juice

2 bags of herbal or decaffeinated green tea

¼ cup gelatin powder

2 tablespoons manuka honey

10 doses CBD isolate or oil-based supplement, either oil-based tincture or nano-liposomal oil

WHAT YOU'LL DO:

1. In a small pan, heat the cherry juice over medium heat.

2. When close to simmering, remove the pan from the heat, add green tea bags, and steep for 4 minutes.

3. Remove the bags. Return the pan to the heat and bring to a simmer. Slowly whisk in the gelatin powder, followed by the honey.

4. Turn the heat to low and continue whisking for another 3–4 minutes. When the gelatin is dissolved, remove the pan from the heat.

5. When the mixture is cooled, stir in the CBD oil.

6. Pour the mixture into molds made from food-grade silicone. Alternatively, you can pour the mixture into a glass baking dish.

7. Allow mixture to harden for two hours in the refrigerator before unmolding. If using a glass baking dish, cut mixture into squares before serving. Wrap in waxed paper and store in an airtight container in the refrigerator for up to two weeks.

WHAT YOU'LL USE IT FOR:

* Insomnia

* Stress

* Anxiety

* Fibromyalgia

* Inflammation

* Immune system enhancement

* Liver disease

* Pain

* Palliative care

* PTS

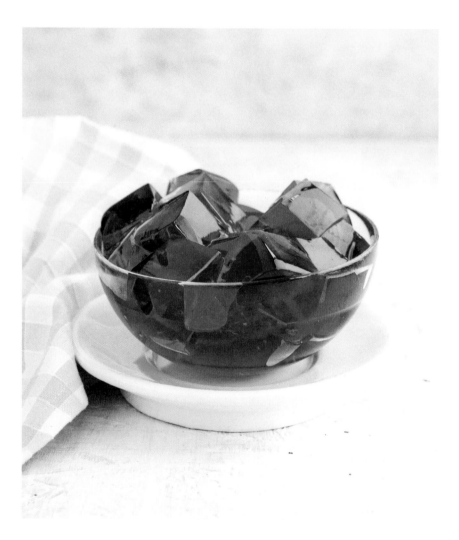

B$_{12}$-BOOSTING HUMMUS

Low levels of vitamin B$_{12}$ are common among vegetarians and are a trigger for depression. Beets and chickpeas are plant-based foods bursting with B$_{12}$, and cumin adds antioxidant and anti-inflammatory benefits.

4 servings

WHAT YOU'LL NEED:

2 small beets

1 clove garlic

1 (12-ounce) can cooked chickpeas, about 1½ cups

3 tablespoons tahini sesame seed paste or tahini

3 tablespoons fresh lemon juice

1½ teaspoons lemon zest

⅓ cup water, used in increments

1½ teaspoons cumin

½ teaspoon sea salt

Fresh ground pepper to taste

A few sprigs of fresh dill or ¼ teaspoon dried dill

4 doses CBD oil-based supplement, either oil-based tincture or nano-liposomal oil

WHAT YOU'LL DO:

1. Boil the beets until tender, about 15 minutes.

2. In the meantime, chop the garlic clove in a food processor; add the chickpeas, tahini, lemon juice, lemon zest, and about half the water, and pulse.

3. Quarter the boiled beets, add to the food processor, and pulse until completely smooth.

4. Add cumin, salt, pepper, and dill, and more water to vary thickness as desired. Blend to incorporate.

5. Blend in the CBD oil.

6. Place in an airtight container and keep chilled in refrigerator for 3–5 days. Serve with your favorite sliced vegetables.

WHAT YOU'LL USE IT FOR:

* Depression

* Stress

* Anxiety

* Inflammation

* Eye health

* Heart health

* Liver health

* Neurodegenerative disease

GHEE-"BUTTERED" POPCORN

Popcorn is one of the most touted snacks for smokers who are trying to quit and need something to do with their hands. Air pop a batch, and add to the thyme-infused ghee and for a snack that engages your hands and calms anxiety. You can also use this ghee in CBD-Ghee and Vegetable Rice (page 172).

3 (5-cup) servings

WHAT YOU'LL NEED:

½ cup (8 tablespoons) high-quality unsalted butter, about 1 stick

1 tablespoon coconut oil

1 teaspoon dried thyme

1 tablespoon olive oil

¾ cup organic popcorn kernels

3 doses CBD oil-based supplement, either oil-based tincture or nano-liposomal oil

Sea salt to taste

WHAT YOU'LL DO:

1. Make the ghee. Cut the unsalted butter into smaller pieces and place in a heavy-bottomed skillet over medium-low heat. Melt the butter and then simmer for 10 minutes, until it foams and starts to boil.

2. Once boiling, push aside the foam and check that the melted butter is clear and golden. If so, allow to cook another minute or so, until the milk solids settle to the bottom and begin to brown. This will add a nutty flavor.

3. Immediately remove the pan from heat. If cooked too long, it will taste burned. Allow the butter to cool for about two minutes.

4. Place a fine mesh strainer, a coffee filter, or cheesecloth over a glass jar, and pour the liquid through it, removing any foam and milk particles. You now have ghee.

5. Place coconut oil, 2 tablespoons ghee, and thyme in a small pan and heat over low heat. Leave heat on for 1 minute after oil has melted, and then turn heat off and cover pan with lid. Set aside.

6. Place olive oil and popcorn in a large pot with a tight-fitting lid, and cook over medium heat, gently shaking the pot regularly. Do not remove the lid.

7. Shake pot continuously once popcorn begins to pop, and continue until popping has slowed significantly or stopped. Turn off heat. Set aside.

8. Add the CBD to thyme-infused oil, and stir.

9. Pour half of the popcorn into a large bowl and drizzle half of the infused ghee over popcorn, gently mixing to coat all popcorn kernels. Pour remaining popcorn into another bowl and cover with remaining infused oil. Mix to coat.

10. Add sea salt to taste over the popcorn. Divide the popcorn between three bowls and enjoy. Makes about 15 cups.

ALTERNATIVE: Remaining ghee can be saved in a closed glass jar in the refrigerator for 3 months. Use it for CBD-Ghee and Vegetable Rice (page 172).

WHAT YOU'LL USE IT FOR:

* Addiction
* Autism

* Stress and anxiety

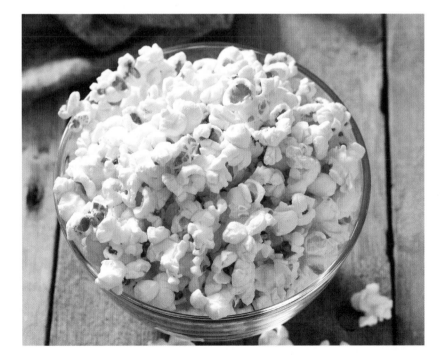

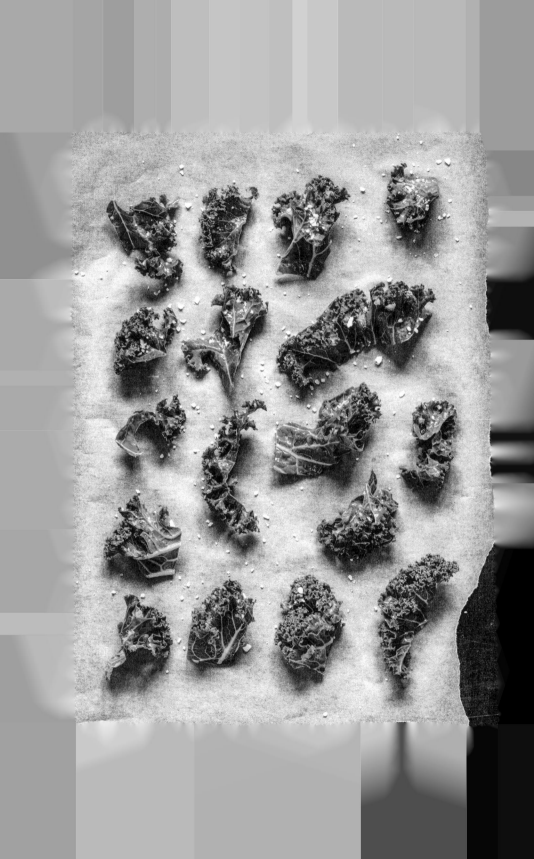

CRUNCHY KALE CHIPS

Add CBD to a crunchy snack like these yummy, flavonoid-rich kale chips, and watch them disappear. Along with hemp seed oil and hemp seeds, CBD is naturally rich in omega-3 fatty acids, essential for brain development and function.

2 servings

WHAT YOU'LL NEED:

6 cups (3 large handfuls) of kale

2 tablespoons extra virgin olive oil

1 teaspoon sea salt

¼ teaspoon garlic or other favorite seasoning

½ teaspoon hemp oil

2 doses CBD oil-based supplement, either oil-based tincture or nano-liposomal oil

2½ teaspoons hemp seeds

WHAT YOU'LL DO:

1. Preheat oven to 350°F.

2. Wash kale thoroughly and use a salad spinner to dry. Place leaves on paper towels and dry further until no moisture remains. It is important that the kale leaves be dry for roasting. Remove stems and break up into pieces.

3. Place kale pieces in a large bowl and drizzle with olive oil, tossing the pieces until they are coated. Season with salt and garlic and toss again to distribute evenly.

4. Arrange kale on an aluminum baking sheet, making sure that pieces are not overcrowded. Bake until crispy but still dark green, about 10–15 minutes. If the leaves brown, they are overcooked. Turn the pieces over halfway through for a balanced bake.

5. While the kale roasts, mix together the hemp and CBD oil in a small bowl. Drizzle the oil over the warm chips just pulled from the oven. Garnish with hemp seeds and serve.

WHAT YOU'LL USE IT FOR:

* Autism (mental focus)

* ADHD (mental focus)

* Epilepsy and seizures

* Immune system support

* Cancer protection

* Neurodegenerative disease (Alzheimer's, mental focus)

FIG CHUTNEY

Five fresh figs carry 90 milligrams of calcium (and a half cup of dried figs a hefty 121 milligrams!), as well as potassium and magnesium, skeletal super-strengtheners. They also have cell-protecting antioxidants, control blood sugar levels, and are rich in fiber. Add CBD and chill this recipe for a luscious, hard-working "medicine."

16 (2-tablespoon) servings or 2 cups

WHAT YOU'LL NEED:

1 tablespoon olive oil

2 shallots, finely diced

1 teaspoon finely chopped thyme

⅓ cup diced apple, peeled

⅓ cup raisins

4 tablespoons honey

1 cup apple cider vinegar

½-inch piece fresh ginger, peeled and minced

Juice and zest of 1 lemon

2 cups dried figs, cut in half

1 teaspoon cinnamon

¼ teaspoon salt

16 doses CBD oil-based supplement, either oil-based tincture or nano-liposomal oil

WHAT YOU'LL DO:

1. In a saucepan, heat the oil.

2. Add the shallots and gently cook on medium-low heat for 2–3 minutes.

3. Add the thyme, apples, raisins, and honey, and stir continuously until the shallots and fruit begin to caramelize, about 5–6 minutes.

4. Add the vinegar, ginger, lemon juice and zest, figs, cinnamon, and salt, and bring the mixture to a boil.

5. Reduce the heat to low and simmer for 20 minutes, stirring frequently.

6. When the figs are thoroughly cooked, remove from heat to cool.

7. When the mixture has cooled, gently stir in the CBD oil.

8. Store the chutney in an airtight container in the refrigerator.

WHAT YOU'LL USE IT FOR:

* Bone health

* Arthritis

* Cancer protection

* Diabetes

* Digestive health (constipation)

* Metabolic syndrome

* Women's health (menopause symptoms: bone loss)

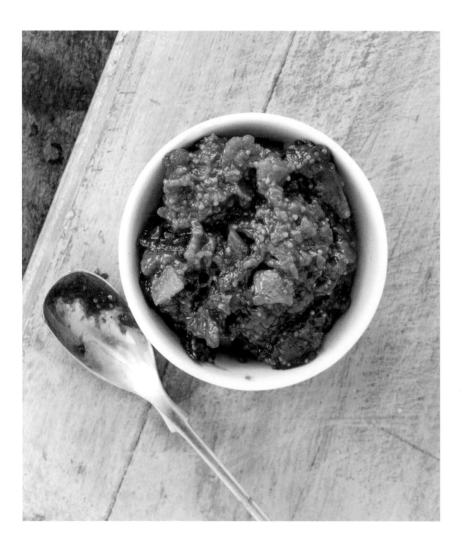

BERRY PROTECTIVE SNACK

Ellagic acid, a powerful antioxidant in strawberries and raspberries, packs an anticancer punch. Research is showing that this plant chemical may fight cancer in a number of ways at once—including by protecting cells from damage, deactivating cancer-causing substances, and inhibiting tumor growth. Add antioxidant dark chocolate and CBD to the mix and you have a delicious disease fighter that has many benefits.

2 servings

WHAT YOU'LL NEED:

2 cups fresh strawberries and raspberries

4 tablespoons dark chocolate, at least 75–80 percent cacao

2 doses CBD oil-based supplement, either oil-based tincture or nano-liposomal oil, flavored with orange, raspberry, peppermint, or other favorite flavor

WHAT YOU'LL DO:

1. Divide the berries between two small bowls.

2. In a double boiler or microwave, melt the dark chocolate. If using a microwave, heat for 30-second intervals. Stir between intervals to ensure even melting.

3. Stir the CBD oil into the chocolate.

4. Drizzle the chocolate mix over the berries. Refrigerate for a half hour, until the chocolate re-hardens, and then serve.

WHAT YOU'LL USE IT FOR:

* Cancer protection

* Asthma

* Depression (antioxidant action)

* Diabetes protection

* Eating disorders (helps lower risk of obesity)

* Epilepsy and seizures

* Heart health

* Immune system protection

* Liver disease

* Metabolic syndrome

* MS and spasticity

* Prostate health

* Psychological disorders

* Stroke and traumatic brain injury

CBD-ALMOND BLISS BALLS

Almonds, like CBD, contain powerful anti-inflammatory and antioxidant benefits. Boosted by coconut's brain-protecting omega-3 fatty acids, this snack brings blissful taste as well as all-around health.

10–12 servings

WHAT YOU'LL NEED:

¾ cups whole almonds

3 tablespoons coconut oil, melted

2 tablespoons manuka honey

10–12 doses CBD oil-based supplement, either oil-based tincture or nano-liposomal oil

½ cup oats

⅓ cup unsweetened shredded coconut

1 tablespoon chia seeds or hemp seeds

3 tablespoons cacao or carob chips

2 teaspoons sesame seeds

WHAT YOU'LL DO:

1. Place almonds in a food processor and pulse until a thick paste forms.

2. In a small bowl, mix together the melted coconut oil, honey, and CBD supplement; then add the mixture to the almond paste, pulsing until the paste becomes smooth nut butter. If not quite smooth enough, add another teaspoon or so of coconut oil.

3. In a large bowl, combine the almond butter, oats, coconut, and chia seeds. Mix until you have a cookie dough consistency. Fold in the cacao or carob chips.

4. Portion a tablespoon of dough at a time and roll into 10–12 golf-size balls.

5. Add sesame seeds to a small dish and dip one side of each ball into the seeds.

6. Store in an airtight container in the refrigerator for 1 week, or in the freezer for a month.

WHAT YOU'LL USE IT FOR:

* Diabetes
* Antiaging
* Cancer protection
* Eating disorders (obesity control)
* Endocrine disorders
* Heart health
* Inflammation

* Stress and anxiety
* Insomnia
* Metabolic syndrome
* MS and spasticity
* Prostate health
* Neurodegenerative disease
  (Alzheimer's)

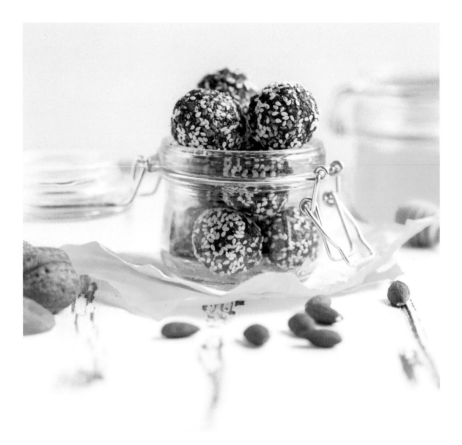

GUACAMOLE DIP

Rich with omega-3 healthy fats and antioxidants and fiber, as well as some seven key vitamins and minerals including B_6, C, E, K, potassium, and folate, avocados have full-body benefits. Heightened by CBD, this fan-favorite dip is a super-health hero.

4 servings

WHAT YOU'LL NEED:

3 medium avocados

3 tablespoons diced red onion

2 small tomatoes, seeded and diced

3 tablespoons chopped fresh cilantro

1 teaspoon minced garlic

Juice of 1 lime, about 2 tablespoons

4 doses CBD oil-based supplement, either oil-based tincture or nano-liposomal oil in neutral flavor

1 teaspoon sea salt

Freshly ground black pepper

Carrots, celery sticks, or pita chips, for serving

WHAT YOU'LL DO:

1. In a bowl, mash the avocados until they reach your desired consistency, either smooth or chunky. Add the onion, tomato, and cilantro.

2. In a separate bowl, whisk together the lime juice and CBD oil. Add the CBD oil mixture to the avocados, gently folding to distribute the CBD oil throughout.

3. Season with sea salt and black pepper to taste. Stir to blend flavors thoroughly. Serve immediately with carrots, celery sticks, or pita chips.

WHAT YOU'LL USE IT FOR:

* Heart health

* Antiaging

* Bone health

* Cancer protection

* Depression (healthy fats for brain food)

* Digestive Issues

* Epilepsy and seizures

* Eye health

* Neurodegenerative disease (protecting brain blood vessels)

* Skin conditions (inner support)

* Psychological disorders

* Stroke and traumatic brain injury

THE THREE Cs

Cocoa, coconut, and CBD may be a winning combination for helping Alzheimer's patients. Products from the cacao plant have long been found to increase blood flow to the brain, and a study in a 2017 issue of *Frontiers of Immunology* shows that it may also be anti-inflammatory, antioxidant, and neuroprotective, possibly lowering production of protein deposits called amyloids that build up in the brains of Alzheimer's patients. Coconut oil has also been observed to improve cognitive function, and it is antibacterial.

12 servings

WHAT YOU'LL NEED:

4 cups unsweetened shredded coconut

1 cup plus 1 tablespoon coconut oil, if needed

1 cup dark cocoa powder

¼ teaspoon cinnamon powder

1 tablespoon raw honey

12 doses CBD oil-based supplement, either oil-based tincture or nano-liposomal oil

WHAT YOU'LL DO:

1. Make the coconut butter. Add shredded coconut to a food processor and blend until smooth, about 20 minutes, stopping to scrape down the sides as needed. If needed, add 1 tablespoon coconut oil during the blending process. Set aside.

2. In a small bowl, mix together the cocoa and cinnamon. Set aside.

3. Melt the coconut oil in a pan over low heat.

4. Gradually add the cocoa mixture to the coconut oil, stirring until it dissolves. Stir in the honey.

5. Line a muffin tin with a dozen paper cups and spoon in the mixture evenly, filling only half of each cup. Refrigerate for 30 minutes so chocolates can set.

6. In a clean saucepan, melt 1 cup of the coconut butter until liquid and remove from heat. Stir in the CBD oil.

7. On top of the solidified chocolate, spoon equal amounts of liquid coconut-CBD butter.

8. Replace in refrigerator until firm, about 30 minutes.

9. Store in the refrigerator in an airtight container for up to 2 weeks, or in the freezer for a month.

ALTERNATIVE: Place coconut butter in an airtight glass jar in a cool, dark place for 2–3 months. It does not need to be refrigerated.

WHAT YOU'LL USE IT FOR:

* Neurodegenerative diseases
* Antiaging
* Depression
* Eating disorders
* Endocrine disorders (restoring hormonal balance)

* Heart health
* Inflammation
* Metabolic syndrome
* Skin conditions (inner support)

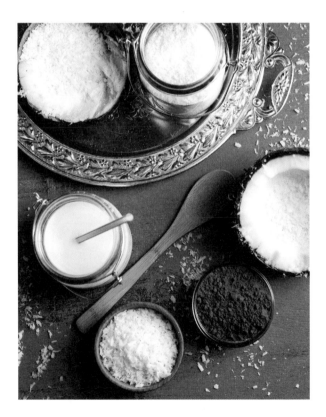

YOGURT POPS

This delicious treat is rich in probiotics that support the gut's healthy bacteria. Research is finding that healthy gut bacteria not only boosts immune function and keeps inflammation in check, but it may also help stabilize emotions. Anti-inflammatory hemp seeds and CBD oil also add to this healthy balance. Adults and kids will welcome this fruity treat and won't worry about mood-spiking refined sugars.

6–8 servings

WHAT YOU'LL NEED:

1 cup plain Greek yogurt

1 cup hemp, almond, or coconut milk

2 tablespoons honey

2 tablespoons hemp seeds

6-8 doses CBD oil-based supplement, either oil-based tincture or nano-liposomal oil

½ cup fresh strawberries, hulled and halved

½ cup fresh blueberries

WHAT YOU'LL DO:

1. Combine the yogurt, milk, honey, hemp seeds, and CBD oil in a blender. Blend until smooth.

2. Add in the fruits and pulse so that fruit is still chunky.

3. Pour the mixture into popsicle molds or paper cups. Cover them with aluminum foil, and punch a popsicle stick through the center of each.

4. Place in the freezer and allow to set for 3–4 hours before enjoying.

WHAT YOU'LL USE IT FOR:

* Psychological disorders

* Asthma

* Bladder health

* Depression

* Digestive issues

* Eating disorders

* Inflammation

* Nausea and vomiting

* PTS

* Stress and anxiety

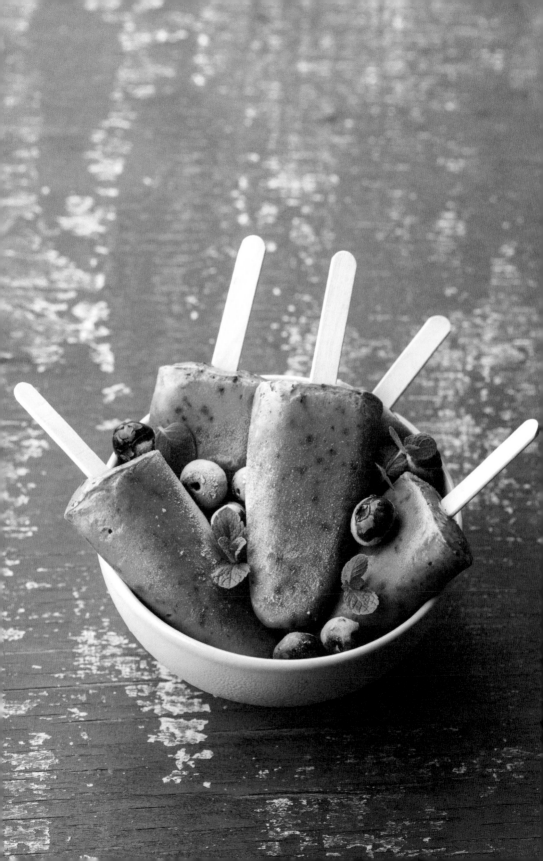

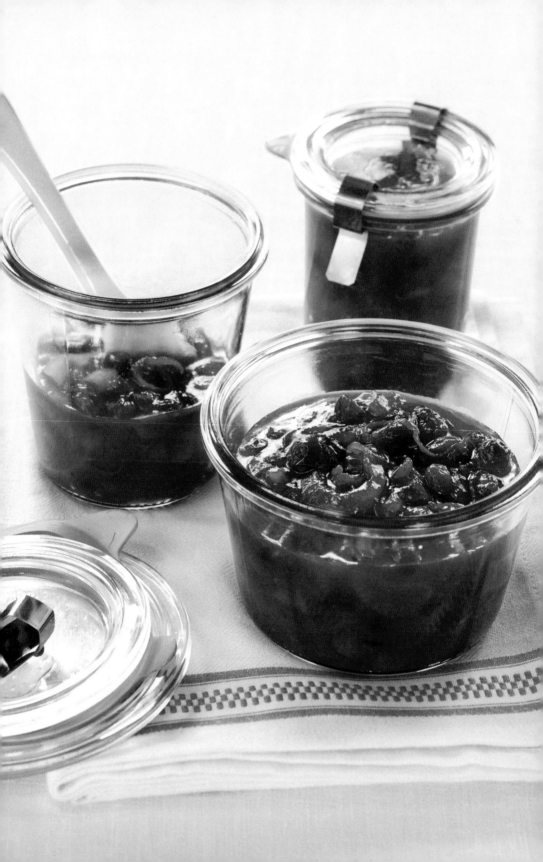

DELICIOUS RAW COMPOTE
Compliments of Deanna Gabriel Vierck

Deanna says: "All the ingredients in this raw compote are antioxidant and cell-protecting, and CBD further enhances the benefits of the fruit's health-promoting flavonoids. In particular, goji berries' plant compounds have been found to help protect the eyes from UV-ray damage and aging."

12 (2-heaping-tablespoon) servings

WHAT YOU'LL NEED:

4 tablespoons unsweetened dried cherries

4 tablespoons dried blueberries

4 tablespoons goji berries

2 tablespoon dried rosehips

1 tablespoon fresh organic orange peels, chopped

12 doses CBD oil-based supplement, either oil-based tincture or nano-liposomal oil

¼–½ teaspoon cinnamon or pumpkin pie spice blend (optional)

½ cup pomegranate juice

WHAT YOU'LL DO:

1. Place the fruit, CBD, and spices in a jar and cover with juice. As the dried fruit absorbs the juice it will expand, so be sure the jar has at least 2–3 inches of space available above the fruit and juice combination.

2. Stir well and cover with a lid. Leave jar on the counter overnight to allow fruit to absorb the liquid. If the fruit still feels a bit dry in the morning, add a small amount of pomegranate juice. If there is an excess of liquid, you can add more dried fruit and allow the mixture to stand for a few more hours for absorption. Store in the refrigerator for up to 1 month. The fruit is delicious on toast, scooped on yogurt, or eaten by the spoonful.

WHAT YOU'LL USE IT FOR:

* Eye health

* Antiaging

* Cancer protection

* Heart health

* Inflammation

* Metabolic syndrome

* MS and spasticity

* Wound healing

SUPER SALMON SALAD AND CBD DRESSING

The majority of kids in two separate ADHD studies in the Netherlands significantly improved focus when eating a diet that was without sugar, wheat, and high-fat meats, but rich in omega-3 foods like salmon, hemp seeds, and hemp seed oil; complex carbs like apples and sweet potatoes; and antioxidant powerhouses like peppers, blueberries, and spinach. Like CBD, these things help balance the calming brain chemicals dopamine and serotonin. This recipe is a boost for other conditions, too.

4 servings

WHAT YOU'LL NEED:

4 pieces of salmon, 4 ounces each

2 tablespoons lemon or lime juice

Salt and pepper to taste

5 cups spinach

1 cup blueberries

1 cup chopped apple

1 cup chopped baked sweet potato

1 cup chopped red or yellow bell pepper

1 teaspoon Dijon mustard

¼ cup balsamic vinegar

1 teaspoon lemon juice

¼ cup hemp seed oil

4 doses CBD oil-based supplement, either oil-based tincture or nano-liposomal oil; try orange-flavored

½ teaspoon fresh chopped rosemary or basil (or ¼ teaspoon dried)

1 teaspoon honey (more to taste if desired)

1 teaspoon crushed hemp seeds or walnuts

NOTE: Deanna says: "Hemp seed oil is extremely fragile. It's ideal to buy it from a refrigerated source and to keep it refrigerated at home. Open and smell immediately after purchase to be sure it's not rancid; return it if it is."

WHAT YOU'LL DO:

1. Preheat the oven to 325°F.

2. Place the salmon, skin side down, in a glass baking dish. Pour lemon juice over the salmon and season to taste with salt and pepper. Bake for 15–20 minutes, until center of the fish is flaky but not overcooked.

3. While salmon is baking, fill a large bowl with the spinach and toss in the blueberries, apple, sweet potato chunks, and bell pepper.

4. In a small bowl, whisk together mustard and vinegar. Add lemon juice and then whisk in hemp seed and CBD oils. Add rosemary or basil and honey and whisk until well combined.

5. Remove the salmon from oven, remove the skin, and baste generously with half the dressing, about ¼ cup. Set aside to cool while plating the dish.

6. Toss the salad in the remaining ¼ cup of dressing, using less if desired, and divide the salad between four plates.

7. Place a warm piece of salmon on top of each salad. Garnish the salad with crushed hemp seeds or walnuts for an extra dose of omega-3s.

WHAT YOU'LL USE IT FOR:

* ADHD
* Asthma
* Autism
* Depression
* Epilepsy and seizures (omega-3 may help control seizures)
* Endocrine disorders
* Eye health (lutein from leafy vegetables)
* Inflammation
* Liver disease
* MS and spasticity
* Neurodegenerative disorders (Alzheimer's)
* Prostate health
* Stress and anxiety
* Psychological disorders
* PTS

CBD-GHEE AND VEGETABLE RICE

Ancient Ayurvedic practice guides patients to avoid raw, cold, or rough foods, and to take in warm, soothing rice, soft vegetables, and mild spices made with a nutrient-rich, nutty-flavored butter called ghee. In ghee, the allergy-prompting dairy, or lactose, has been removed. Studies in India show that ghee has appetite-restoring powers without the cholesterol concerns of other oils. CBD enhances its benefits.

4 (¼-cup) servings

WHAT YOU'LL NEED:

½ cup (8 tablespoons) high-quality unsalted butter, about 1 stick

4 doses CBD oil-based supplement, either oil-based tincture or nano-liposomal oil

1⅓ cup water, divided

¼ cup raw basmati rice (yields ¾ cup cooked rice)

Pinch salt

1 cup raw vegetables, diced, such as parsnips, beets, turnips, sweet potato, squash, carrots, or broccoli florets

¼ teaspoon cinnamon

¼ teaspoon cumin

WHAT YOU'LL DO:

1. Make the ghee. Cut the unsalted butter into smaller pieces and place in a heavy-bottomed skillet. Melt the butter and then simmer for 10 minutes, until it foams and starts to boil.

2. Once boiling, push aside the foam and check that the melted butter is clear and golden. If so, allow to cook for a bit longer until the milk solids settle to the bottom and begin to brown. This will add a nutty flavor.

3. Immediately remove the pan from heat. If cooked too long, it will taste burned. Allow the butter to cool for about two minutes.

4. Place a fine mesh strainer, a coffee filter, or cheesecloth over a glass jar, and pour the liquid through it, removing any foam and milk particles. You now have ghee.

5. Stir in the CBD oil, mixing thoroughly. Close the lid and refrigerate when finished using.

6. Make the vegetable rice. In a pan, boil ⅓ cup water and a pinch of salt. Once boiling, add the basmati rice, lower the heat, and steam until the rice is soft and the water evaporates, about 15 minutes.

7. In a separate pan, use 1 cup water to steam the vegetable mix until soft; strain the water, and fold the vegetables into the warm rice.

8. Stir the cinnamon and cumin into the rice. Add 2 tablespoons ghee and gently stir until evenly distributed throughout the rice-vegetable mixture. Divide among four plates and serve. Reheat leftovers, as needed.

ALTERNATIVE: Use coconut oil instead of butter. Skip to step 5 and mix the coconut oil with the CBD oil. Proceed with the recipe.

WHAT YOU'LL USE IT FOR:

* Eating disorders (anorexia and cachexia)

* Autism (if coconut oil replaces CBD-ghee)

* Endocrine disorder (if coconut oil replaces CBD-ghee)

* Eye health (lutein from yellow vegetables in rice)

* Cancer and chemotherapy (reduces appetite loss)

* Diabetes

* Liver health

* Nausea and vomiting (for recovery)

* Metabolic syndrome

* Palliative care

* Prostate health

KALE AND SEAWEED SALAD

Compliments of Amy Ellis, Color Cuisine (www.colorcuisine.co)

The ocean is an incredible source of nutritious sea vegetables packed with iodine for thyroid health. In fact, your thyroid has the only cells that absorb iodine in order to make key hormones to keep your body humming along. Vegetables like kale and seaweed are also rich in calcium, potassium, and copper.

4 servings

WHAT YOU'LL NEED:

1 tablespoon avocado oil

1 shallot, chopped

1 clove garlic, minced

1–2 tablespoons minced ginger

1 head kale, roughly chopped

¼ cup arame seaweed, soaked and drained

1 tablespoon coconut aminos

2 teaspoons toasted sesame oil

1 tablespoon black or white sesame seeds

4 doses CBD oil-based supplement, either oil-based tincture or nano-liposomal oil

WHAT YOU'LL DO:

1. In a skillet, heat avocado oil over medium heat. Add shallots, garlic, and ginger and sauté for 3 minutes.

2. Add the kale and sauté for 2 minutes more.

3. Turn off the heat and remove the skillet from the heat. Add the seaweed, coconut aminos, sesame oil and seeds, and CBD oil. Toss to combine and then serve.

WHAT YOU'LL USE IT FOR:

* Endocrine disorders

* Bone health

* Cancer protection

* Digestive issues

* MS and spasticity

* Women's health (PMS and Menopause)

SAGE CHICKEN AND APPLES

According to the Epilepsy Foundation, research since the 1920s has measured the effect of diet on seizures. Statistics consistently show that a natural, whole foods diet that eliminates sugar and alcohol and is rich in protein, complex carbohydrates (like fruits, vegetables, and whole grains), and omega-3 fats may help lower the number of seizures. Each of these foods plays a key part in building and maintaining healthy brain cells.

4 servings

WHAT YOU'LL NEED:

2 tablespoons finely minced fresh sage (use a coffee grinder to reach a fine consistency)

½ teaspoon salt

¼ teaspoon black pepper

2 large boneless, skinless chicken breasts

2 tablespoons extra-virgin olive oil

1 medium onion, thinly sliced

2 medium apples, peeled, cored, and thinly sliced

½ teaspoon cinnamon

2 tablespoons apple cider vinegar

Cooked whole grain couscous, brown rice, or cauliflower rice, for serving

1½ tablespoons CBD-infused ghee (see steps 1–4 on page 154)

WHAT YOU'LL DO:

1. In a small dish, mix together 1 tablespoon sage with the salt and pepper; then massage the herb mix into the chicken breasts. Cut each breast into ¼-inch-wide strips. Set aside.

2. In a large skillet, heat the olive oil over medium-high heat.

3. Add the onion, apple slices, and cinnamon and sauté for 3–4 minutes, until lightly browned.

4. Move the apples and onions to the perimeter of the pan. Add the chicken strips to the center of the pan. Brown the chicken strips, about 4 minutes on each side.

5. While the chicken cooks, mix together the vinegar and remaining sage in a small dish. Pour vinegar into pan and stir to distribute evenly.

6. Reduce the heat to medium and continue cooking the chicken another 3–4 minutes, until it is cooked through.

7. Dish up the chicken, apples, and onion while warm over four bowls of whole grain couscous, brown rice, or cauliflower rice.

8. Gently heat the CBD-ghee in a saucepan over low heat. Drizzle the butter over each bowl and serve.

WHAT YOU'LL USE IT FOR:

* Epilepsy and seizure disorders
* ADHD
* Autism
* MS and spasticity
* Neurodegenerative disorders (Alzheimer's)

OAT EXTRAVAGANZA

Inside each grain of modest breakfast cereal are the mighty healing powers of calcium, zinc, iron, B vitamins, and other nutrients. Oats also help limit blood lipids, or fats, that damage arteries and raise blood pressure. Use the steel-cut variety to get the benefits of the entire oat kernel.

2 servings

WHAT YOU'LL NEED:

½ cup steel-cut oats

1½ cups water

1 medium apple with skin on, cored and chopped

1 teaspoon minced fresh ginger

1 tablespoon raisins

¼ cup walnut pieces

1 teaspoon ground cinnamon, nutmeg, or pumpkin pie spice

1 tablespoon hemp seeds

2 tablespoons CBD-infused ghee (see steps 1–4 on page 154)

2 tablespoons plain nonfat Greek yogurt

WHAT YOU'LL DO:

1. In a saucepan, bring the water to a boil over high heat then lower to a simmer. Add the oats, apple, and ginger, stirring occasionally as the oats thicken, about 25 minutes.

2. Immediately remove from heat and stir in the spice of choice, raisins, and walnuts. Stir in the hemp seeds; then spoon the oats into two bowls.

3. Stir a tablespoon of CBD-infused ghee into each serving. Top with a tablespoon of yogurt and serve.

ALTERNATIVE: Substitute coconut oil for CBD-infused ghee, and stir in two doses of CBD oil. Or top each bowl with a scoop of Delicious Raw Compote (page 169).

WHAT YOU'LL USE IT FOR:

* Metabolic syndrome

* Bone health (calcium)

* Heart health

* Diabetes

* MS andspasticity (if coconut oil or raw compote is used)

* Stroke prevention

LUSCIOUS TOMATO-WALNUT PESTO

Tomatoes are packed with lycopene, a cell-protecting antioxidant that helps fight cancer. They also have other heart- and skin-protecting qualities. Add nutritious hemp seeds and CBD oil for more benefits.

4–6 servings

WHAT YOU'LL NEED:

4 cups chopped tomatoes, peeled and seeded

2 cloves garlic, minced

½ cup packed fresh basil leaves

2 tablespoons walnut pieces

2 tablespoons hemp seeds

½ cup hemp seed oil

2 teaspoons balsamic vinegar

½ teaspoon oregano

½ teaspoon sea salt

A dash of black pepper

½ cup freshly grated Parmesan cheese

4 doses CBD oil-based supplement, either oil-based tincture or nano-liposomal oil

Spaghetti squash, pasta, or spinach noodles, for serving

WHAT YOU'LL DO:

1. In a blender, puree all the ingredients except the Parmesan cheese, CBD oil, and spaghetti squash or pasta.

2. When the mixture is smooth, add the cheese and blend just enough so that it is combined.

3. Add the CBD oil and pulse to combine.

4. Top a dish of spaghetti squash or your favorite pasta with pesto. Spinach noodles are a nutrient-rich alternative.

WHAT YOU'LL USE IT FOR:

* Prostate health

* Cancer protection

* Depression (omega-3)

* Endocrine disorders

* Heart health

* Skin protection (inner support)

* MS and spasticity

* Psychological disorders (omega-3)

* Stroke and traumatic brain injury (omega-3)

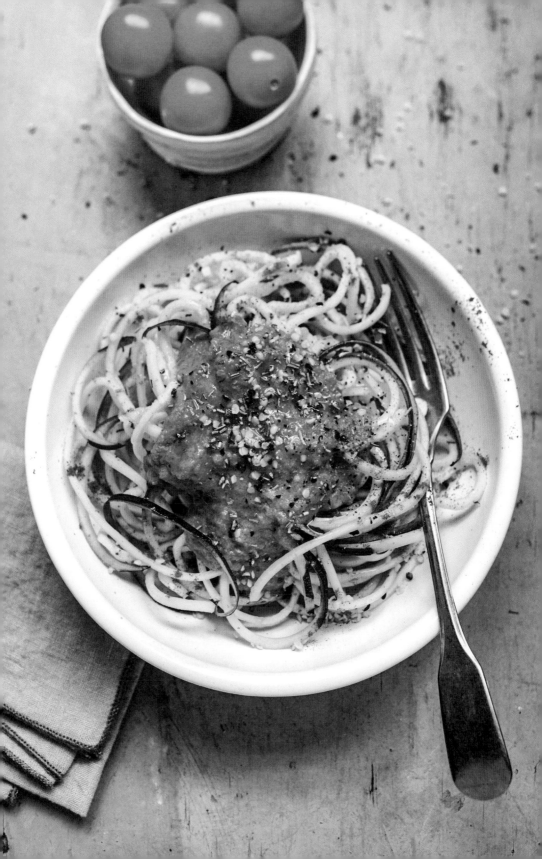

SPINACH CURRY

This easy dish combines many of the fragrant and antioxidant herbs that make up curry, including curcumin-rich turmeric and vitamin E–rich spinach. CBD and hemp seeds add healthful omega-3s and other benefits.

Servings: 4 (1-cup) servings or 8 (½-cup) servings

WHAT YOU'LL NEED:

2 tablespoons olive oil

1 medium onion, chopped

1 medium tomato, chopped

4 cloves garlic, minced

1 tablespoon chopped fresh ginger root

1 teaspoon turmeric

2 teaspoons coriander

¼ teaspoon cumin

¼ teaspoon black pepper (use more or less as desired)

½ teaspoon cinnamon

1 cup fresh cilantro, washed and destemmed

1 cup chicken stock, divided

16 ounces fresh baby spinach, washed and dried

½ teaspoon salt (use more or less as desired)

1 (about 15-ounce) can chickpeas, rinsed and drained

1 cup plain Greek yogurt (use more as needed)

4–8 doses CBD oil-based supplement, either oil-based tincture or nano-liposomal oil

2 tablespoons hemps seeds

WHAT YOU'LL DO:

1. In a large pan over medium heat, add olive oil, and sauté onion, tomato, garlic, and ginger, about 3–5 minutes.

2. Add turmeric, coriander, cumin, black pepper, cinnamon, and cilantro while continuing to sauté.

3. Pour ½ cup chicken stock into the pan and stir. Add the spinach. Turn the heat to medium low, stir, and cover for about 5 minutes.

4. When the spinach has wilted, remove the pan from the heat and allow spinach to cool for 5 minutes.

5. In a blender, blend the spinach mixture until smooth, adding remaining chicken stock to thin the mixture, as needed.

6. Return the mixture to the pan and turn heat back to medium. Stir in the salt and chickpeas, and bring to a simmer. Fold ½ cup yogurt into the sauce.

7. In a separate small bowl, mix the remaining ½ cup yogurt with the CBD oil.

8. Divide the curry among four separate bowls and top each bowl with 2 tablespoons CBD-enriched yogurt. If serving eight, use 1 tablespoon of yogurt for each. Garnish with hemp seeds and serve with rice.

ALTERNATIVE: Instead of adding the final CBD-enriched dollop of yogurt, you can simply stir a dose of CBD oil into each serving.

WHAT YOU'LL USE IT FOR:

* Stroke and traumatic brain injury
* Cancer protection
* Depression
* Neurodegenerative diseases (Alzheimer's)
* Psychological concerns

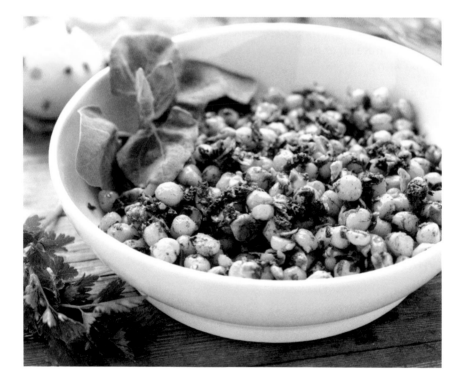

ANTIAGING SERUM

CBD, rosehip oil, and hemp seed oil are a powerful antioxidant triumvirate that fights cell damage, along with the wrinkles and loss of elasticity that come with aging. Lavender essential oil also offers moisturizing and anti-inflammatory properties.

10 (⅛-teaspoon or ½-dropperful) applications

WHAT YOU'LL NEED:

¼ teaspoon hemp seed oil

8 doses CBD oil-based tincture (Start with ½ dropper, 15 drops, or ⅛ teaspoon of a 250-mg/ounce supplement for a 4-mg dose, or for a total of 4 dropperfuls for 8 doses. Select a neutral-scented CBD so it doesn't irritate your skin.)

1 drop lavender essential oil

1 serving of rosehip oil, 2–4 drops per serving (I suggest 4 drops)

WHAT YOU'LL DO:

1. Combine the ingredients in a small bowl and stir with a chopstick.

2. Cover the bowl with plastic and store in a dark, cool place for 5 days.

3. Each morning, massage ⅛ teaspoon into your face and neck for day-long moisturizing with a glow. Apply again before bedtime to reinforce the skin-restoring powers of sleep.

ALTERNATIVE: If you decide to make a bigger batch (about five times the amount), store the serum in a 1-ounce dropper bottle. Keep the bottle in a dark, cool place.

WHAT YOU'LL USE IT FOR:

* Antiaging

* Arthritis

* Inflammation (topical)

* Skin conditions (psoriasis, eczema)

* Wound healing (for scabbed wounds; for scar prevention)

CBD-GINGER-ALOE ARTHRITIS PASTE

Ginger and aloe are time-honored remedies for inflamed joints and muscles, especially popular in Indian Ayurvedic medicine. This recipe is simple but effective on its own; and a CBD addition can add a boost of relief.

1 application

WHAT YOU'LL NEED:

¼ cup fresh grated ginger

1 cup water

1 tablespoon aloe gel

1 dose CBD oil-based tincture (Start with ⅛ teaspoon or ½ dropper or 15 drops of a

250-mg/ounce CBD supplement to get one 4-mg dose of CBD per serving.)

Cheesecloth or other clean cloth (see alternative below)

WHAT YOU'LL DO:

1. In a pan over low heat, mix together the ginger and water. Simmer until the water has nearly disappeared, about 15–20 minutes.

2. Remove the pan from the heat. Transfer the warm ginger into a small bowl.

3. Mix together with the aloe to form a paste.

4. Add the CBD oil.

5. Spread the mixture over the inflamed joint.

6. Cover with a clean cloth. Rest for 15 minutes to a half hour, and then wash away.

ALTERNATIVE: Spread the mixture over the cloth and push down on it to saturate the cloth. Then apply the cloth to the joint.

CAUTION: The direct application with ginger may sting at first, but it usually subsides quickly. Try a small sample on your skin without CBD oil. If you tolerate it, add the CBD to the recipe. If it burns, quickly wash it off.

WHAT YOU'LL USE IT FOR:

* Arthritis

* Inflammation (muscle and joint)

* Fibromyalgia

* Lyme disease (joint inflammation)

DOUBLE ACTION: CBD-LAVENDER AROMATHERAPY AND MASSAGE

Inhaling steam with lavender can help quickly open bronchial airways and relieve mucus buildup. This recipe also makes a soothing rub to massage into the chest to help keep airways open and relieve spasms.

1 application

WHAT YOU'LL NEED:

Vaporizer

Sterile water

10 drops lavender essential oil, divided

1 tablespoon hemp seed oil

1 dose CBD oil-based tincture (Start with ⅛ teaspoon, ½ dropper, or 15 drops of a 250-mg/ounce supplement for a 4-mg dose per application.)

WHAT YOU'LL DO:

1. Fill the vaporizer with sterile water.

2. Add 5 drops of lavender essential oil and start the vaporizer.

3. In a small, clean dish, mix together the hemp seed oil, the CBD oil, and 5 remaining drops of lavender.

4. Massage the mixture into your chest.

5. Relax in a comfortable position; use the vaporizer at night during sleep to help keep airways open.

ALTERNATIVE: To soothe from within, remove the lavender essential oil from the chest rub recipe and swallow the mixture. For immediate relief from breathlessness and an anxiety attack, use a CBD vaporizer pen. Start slowly, with a small amount, to avoid allergic reaction.

NOTE: Do not give up your prescriptive inhaler in place of alternative remedies.

WHAT YOU'LL USE IT FOR:

* Asthma

* Inflammation (cough and cold)

* Headache

* Women's conditions (PMS cramps)

PAIN-CALMING MASSAGE OIL

This CBD-rich Saint John's wort oil, combined with calming lavender and pain-fighting peppermint essential oils, has the potential to address the inflammation and discomfort of fibromyalgia, arthritis, or even sunburn.

16 (1-tablespoon) applications

WHAT YOU'LL NEED:

½ cup fresh Saint John's wort flower buds

1 cup olive oil

5 drops lavender essential oil

5 drops peppermint essential oil

16 doses CBD alcohol- or oil-based tincture (Start with ⅛ teaspoon, ½ dropper, or 15 drops of a 250-mg/ounce supplement for a 4-mg dose per 1 tablespoon [4 dropper] application of the oil.)

WHAT YOU'LL DO:

1. Add the flower buds to a glass jar.

2. Cover the herb fully with olive oil and secure the jar's lid tightly.

3. Place the jar in the sunlight for about 3 weeks, shaking it often. The olive oil will turn red as the flower glands release their oils.

4. Using a strainer or cheesecloth, strain out the Saint John's wort flower buds and transfer the oil into a clean jar. Mix in the lavender and peppermint essential oil. Add the CBD oil.

5. Tightly cap the jar and shake vigorously to combine the healing oils. While using, store in a dark, cool place for up to 6 months. Use the mixture topically, as needed.

CAUTION: This recipe is for topical application. Do not take internally.

WHAT YOU'LL USE IT FOR:

* Fibromyalgia

* Arthritis

* Headache

* Inflammation

* Lyme disease (joint pain)

* Pain (muscle and joint)

* Palliative care

* Women's health

* Wound care (bruising)

CBD FOOT BATH BOMBS

Compliments of Ashlee Sarkozy, owner, Botanical Roots, a natural skin care company (www.BotanicalRoots.com)

Deep rest and nourishing herbs can be part of a whole-body healing regimen for those with Lyme disease, believe clinical herbalists Katja Swift and Ryn Midura of the Commonwealth Center for Holistic Herbalism in Boston, Massachusetts. In the recipe below, from Ashlee Sarkozy of Botanical Roots, in Denver, Colorado, essential oils and CBD in a foot bath bomb help soothe inflammation.

6 applications (makes 12 foot bath bombs; use 2 at a time)

WHAT YOU'LL NEED:

1 cup baking soda

½ cup organic cornstarch

1 cup citric acid (can be found online or where you'd find canning supplies)

2 tablespoons Epsom salt

½ cup organic olive, avocado, or melted coconut oil

25 drops lavender essential oil

8 drops peppermint essential oil

5 drops spearmint essential oil

6 doses CBD oil-based tincture (Start with ⅛ teaspoon, ½ dropper, or 15 drops of a 250-mg/ounce supplement for a 4-mg dose per 2 foot bath bombs, for a total of 3 dropperfuls. Titrate up or down as you wish.)

Molds, such as silicone ice cube trays or muffin tins

WHAT YOU'LL DO:

1. Mix the baking soda, cornstarch, citric acid, and Epsom salt together in a bowl.

2. In a separate bowl, add the oil, essential oils, and CBD. Mix well.

3. Very slowly add the oil mixture to the dry ingredients and mix well, using either a spoon or your hands. You will want the mixture to be like damp sand. It should stick together when pressed.

4. Pack the mixture tightly into molds.

5. Leave in molds overnight; empty the molds and store in a glass container for up to six months.

NOTE: This recipe uses lavender, peppermint, and spearmint for their relaxing yet uplifting qualities; but to assist with the "brain fog" of Lyme disease, consider frankincense, lemon, and vetiver instead.

WHAT YOU'LL USE IT FOR:

* Lyme disease
* Addiction (anxiety of withdrawal)
* Insomnia
* Palliative care

* PTS
* Stress and anxiety
* Women's health

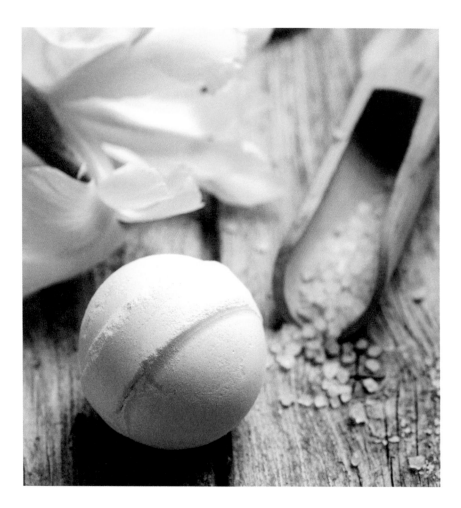

PEPPERY PAIN RELIEF SALVE

For nagging back, neck, migraine, or arthritis pain, try this warming treatment with cayenne pepper. Rich in capsaicin, this active component interrupts the nerves' ability to transmit pain signals between inflamed areas and your brain. While creating a warming sensation, it also blots out discomfort. If you're using it for migraine, rub it into your shoulders and neck, and be careful to keep it away from your eyes.

48 (2-teaspoon) applications

WHAT YOU'LL NEED:

1 cup coconut oil

1 cup extra virgin olive oil

3 tablespoons beeswax

12 drops Roman chamomile or lavender essential oil

¼ teaspoon cayenne pepper

1 dose CBD oil-based tincture (Start with ⅛ teaspoon or ½ dropper of a 250-mg/ounce supplement for a 4-mg dose per application.)

WHAT YOU'LL DO:

1. In a pan over low heat, warm the coconut oil, olive oil, and beeswax, stirring until it has a creamy but not fully solid texture.

2. Remove the pan from the heat and quickly stir in the Roman chamomile essential oil.

3. Pour the mixture into a single pint glass container with a lid and let cool.

4. When the mixture has cooled, cap the jar and store in a dark, cool place.

5. For each application, add 2 teaspoons of the oil mixture into a small bowl.

6. Blend in the cayenne pepper; then add the drops of CBD oil.

7. Massage the salve into shoulders, neck, and lower back. Get help for hard-to-reach places.

ALTERNATIVE: For a very simple fix, mix ¼ teaspoon cayenne powder and a dose of CBD oil into 2 teaspoons of your favorite hand or body cream.

WHAT YOU'LL USE IT FOR:

* Pain

* Arthritis

* Fibromyalgia

* Headache

* Inflammation

* Women's health (PMS abdominal pain)

* Wound care (for pain from healing, not open wounds)

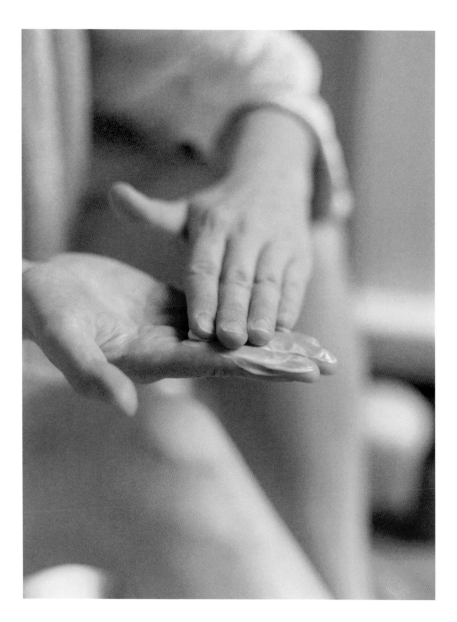

CBD-LAVENDER-COLLOIDAL OAT IMMERSION

Applied topically, oats moisturize the skin and decrease itching and inflammation. Lavender and CBD are also anti-inflammatory and soothing. This recipe makes for a relaxing, immersive bath.

1 application

WHAT YOU'LL NEED:

2–3 cups regular or colloidal oats

15 drops lavender essential oil

Clean sock

1 dose CBD oil-based tincture (Start with ⅜ teaspoon or 1½ droppers of a 250-mg/ounce supplement for a 12-mg dose—larger than usual because it will dissolve in a large tub of water.)

WHAT YOU'LL DO:

1. If using regular oats, pour them into a food processor, coffee grinder, or blender, and blend to a powder. This turns them into colloidal oats.

2. In a bowl, mix the oats, lavender oil, and CBD oil until well combined.

3. Pour the oats into a sock to contain the particles and ease cleanup. Be sure to knot the sock at the top.

4. Fill a tub with warm water, placing the sock beneath the spout so the running water disperses the contents of the sock.

5. Climb in and soak for at least 15 minutes, without soap, which dries and irritates the skin. Gently rub the sock along arms, legs, and torso, squeezing it like a sponge to coat the skin with the soothing oat extract.

6. Pat dry with a clean towel. Do not rub dry.

ALTERNATIVE: Use the oatmeal sock in a foot bath and rub the sock against your aching feet and ankles. If using a small tub for a foot bath, cut the CBD oil-based tincture in half.

WHAT YOU'LL USE IT FOR:

* Palliative care
* Bladder health (for UTI)
* Inflammation
* Fibromyalgia

* Pain
* Skin conditions
* Stress and anxiety
* Women's health

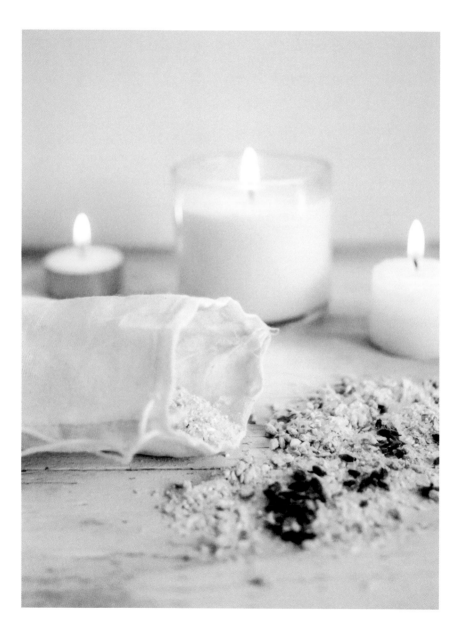

HEMP SEED OIL SKIN SOOTHER

Hemp seed oil contributes anti-inflammatory and healing properties. Coconut oil works as an antibacterial, and tea tree oil contains terpenes that allow it to deliver both antibacterial and soothing properties. CBD adds to these effects. Without tea tree, this recipe can soothe outbreaks of eczema. With tea tree, it targets acne.

24 (½-teaspoon) applications

WHAT YOU'LL NEED:

2 teaspoons coconut oil

¼ cup hemp seed oil

24 doses CBD oil-based tincture (Start with ⅛ teaspoon or ½ dropper of a 250-mg/ounce supplement for a 4-mg dose per application, for a total of 12 dropperfuls.)

5–10 drops tea tree essential oil (Start with 5 drops and test on skin; add more as tolerated.)

WHAT YOU'LL DO:

1. In a microwave-safe dish, heat the coconut oil in the microwave until completely melted, using 30-second intervals.

2. Pour the coconut oil into a small dish. Add the hemp seed oil and stir. Stir in the CBD oil and tea tree oil.

3. Smooth the mixture over the affected area. Store the remaining mixture in a glass jar in a dark, cool place for six months.

ALTERNATIVE: Apply directly onto acne before bedtime. In the morning, wash away with cool water.

WHAT YOU'LL USE IT FOR:

* Skin conditions

* Antibiotic-resistant bacterial infection

* Inflammation (topical)

* Wounds

CRAMP-SOOTHING CASTOR PACK

While many think of castor oil as a laxative, it has long been used in naturopathic medicine to treat pain and inflammation from menstrual cramps, uterine fibroids, and ovarian cysts. Cinnamon and lavender essential oil and CBD support castor oil's efforts in this simple home remedy.

1 application

WHAT YOU'LL NEED:

½ cup castor oil

3 drops lavender essential oil

3 drops cinnamon essential oil

1 dose CBD oil-based tincture (Start with ⅛ teaspoon or ½ dropper of a 250-mg/ounce supplement for a 4-mg dose for each application.)

Large cotton flannel cloth, about 2 feet by 2 feet

Plastic wrap

Hot water bottle

Large towel

WHAT YOU'LL DO:

1. In a bowl, mix together the castor oil, lavender, cinnamon, and CBD oil.

2. Fold the cloth into two or three layers and dip it into the castor oil mixture, creating a pack.

3. Lie in a comfortable position and apply the pack to your abdomen.

4. Cover it with a piece of plastic wrap and settle the hot water bottle on top.

5. With the large towel, cover the hot water bottle and tuck the towel beneath your buttocks to hold in the warmth close to your body.

6. Close your eyes for 40 minutes to an hour as cramping eases.

WHAT YOU'LL USE IT FOR:

* Women's health (PMS abdominal cramps and other discomfort)

* Inflammation

* Arthritis

* Fibromyalgia

* Lyme disease

* Pain management

MANUKA HONEY SALVE

In 2007, the U.S. Food and Drug Administration backed the use of manuka honey—a product of New Zealand—for wound-treating due to its success as a bacteria and inflammation fighter. Aloe echoes its healing benefits, and the two make a dynamic duo. Their early combined use for treating wounds was recorded by ancient Roman naturalist Pliny the Elder. CBD jumps in with similar benefits, along with pain-relieving powers. You can try this easy salve on small first-degree burns, too.

8 (¼-teaspoon) applications

WHAT YOU'LL NEED:

1 teaspoon aloe vera gel, either fresh from the plant or a commercial product that is at least 99 percent aloe vera

1 teaspoon manuka honey

1 dose CBD oil-based tincture (Start with ⅛ teaspoon or ½ dropper of a 250-mg/ounce CBD supplement to get a 4-mg dose of CBD for each application. Titrate up or down as needed.)

WHAT YOU'LL DO:

1. In a small bowl, blend the aloe gel and honey; stir in the CBD oil.

2. Spread the balm over the washed wound and store the remainder in a covered container in the refrigerator. Use the mixture within a week.

3. Repeat as needed throughout the day.

TIP: You can run cool water over the burn to start the cooling process while mixing the salve.

WHAT YOU'LL USE IT FOR:

* Wounds

* Antibiotic-resistant bacterial infection

* Inflammation

* Pain and chronic pain

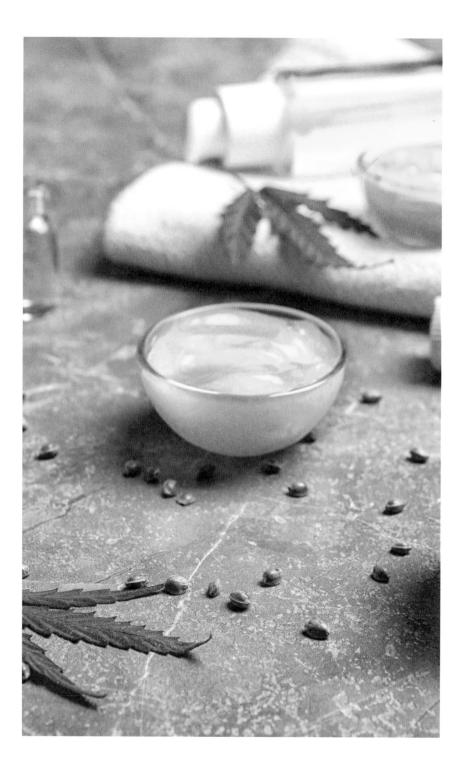

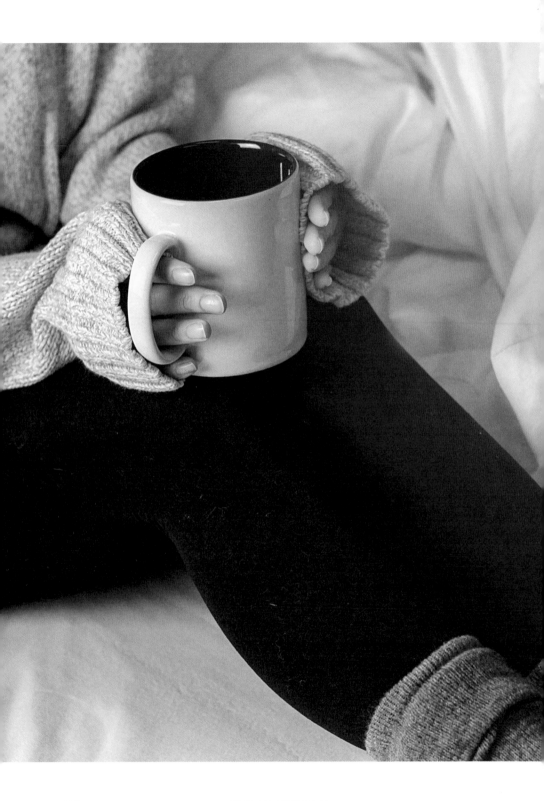

CBD HANDBOOK

CBD-OAT RELIEF

Oats are chock-full of thiamin and pantothenic acid, which work together to soothe nerves. CBD heightens the effect.

1 serving

WHAT YOU'LL NEED:

1 tablespoon rolled or steel-cut oats

1 cup water

1 dose CBD oil-based supplement, either oil-based tincture or nano-liposomal oil

WHAT YOU'LL DO:

1. Place the water and oats in a pan and bring water to a boil.

2. Once boiling, lower the heat and allow it to simmer for 15 minutes.

3. Using a strainer, separate the liquid and oats. Be sure to strain the liquid into a cup. Discard the oats.

4. Add the CBD to the creamy liquid and sip.

WHAT YOU'LL USE IT FOR:

* Anxiety

* Stress

* ADHD

* Nausea and vomiting

* PTS

* Psychological disorders

* Palliative care

FENNEL DIGESTIF

A bitter digestif aids in digestion after a meal, relieving gas and bloating caused by certain foods. Fennel is a go-to for heartburn, bloating, and intestinal gas; it may relax the colon and decrease secretions of the respiratory tract. Combined with CBD's anti-inflammatory and anti-GERD benefits, it sets up the diner for a comfortable after-dinner experience.

16 (2-tablespoon) servings

WHAT YOU'LL NEED:

1 tablespoon fennel seeds

¼ cup leafy fennel stalk

2 cups vodka

Agave nectar or honey

10 drops lavender or chamomile essential oil 16 doses CBD alcohol- or oil-based supplement, either oil-based tincture or nano-liposomal oil

WHAT YOU'LL DO:

1. Place the fennel seeds and stalks in a glass quart jar. Add the vodka, covering the fennel with at least 1 inch of vodka above the herb.

2. Cap the mixture tightly, shake well, and allow it to steep at room temperature for at least one week.

3. After steeping is complete, strain out the herb and measure the remaining liquid.

4. Divide the liquid's measure in half and add the same amount of agave nectar. For example, if the liquid measures 1 cup, you would add ½ cup agave. Stir the agave thoroughly.

5. Add the essential oil and CBD and shake thoroughly. Sip 2 tablespoons alone, or add to sparkling water or a cup of warm water. Store the digestif in the freezer.

ALTERNATIVE: Deanna says: "Lavender and chamomile both offer additional bitters to boost digestive function, and both herbs soothe the nervous system—there are so many nerves throughout the digestive system! This recipe is mostly alcohol based, so if you bump a serving up to ¼ cup, it turns into a delicious cocktail."

WHAT YOU'LL USE IT FOR:

* Digestive issues
* Inflammation
* Nausea and vomiting (If recipe is diluted in flat or sparkling water)
* Stress and anxiety
* Women's health (bloating during PMS)

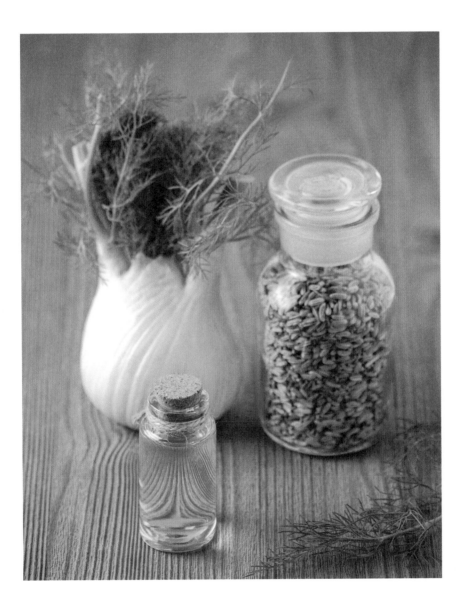

ELDERBERRY SYRUP
Compliments of Deanna Gabriel Vierck

Elderberries offer nutritional boosts by providing vitamins C and A, as well as antioxidants. There are a number of studies that indicate consuming elderberries during cold and flu season can offer enough immune boost to help you avoid illness or shorten the duration of common seasonal infections.

32 (2-tablespoon) servings or 64 (1-tablespoon) servings

WHAT YOU'LL NEED:

2 cups elderberries

1 teaspoon cinnamon chips

1 teaspoon cardamom hulls

1 teaspoon dried ginger root pieces

1 tablespoon of echinacea root (optional)

4 cups water

Honey (equal to volume of strained tea)

32 doses CBD isolate or oil-based supplement, either oil-based tincture or nano-liposomal oil

WHAT YOU'LL DO:

1. Place the elderberries, cinnamon chips, cardamom hulls, and dried ginger root and echinacea root in a saucepan and cover with water.

2. Bring the mixture to a gentle boil and then reduce heat. Simmer for 30–40 minutes, stirring occasionally. Remove from the heat and let cool.

3. Once mixture is cool enough to work with, mash berries with a large spoon or potato masher.

4. Strain tea through a fine mesh strainer or cheesecloth over a jar or pitcher. Measure the remaining liquid.

5. Add the same amount of honey to the tea. For example, if the liquid measures 1 cup, you would add 1 cup honey. Stir the honey thoroughly.

6. Pour elderberry syrup into a large mason jar or glass. Stir in the CBD supplement.

7. Store the syrup in amber bottles in the fridge for 6 months.

ALTERNATIVE: Place mashed herbs into a glass mason jar and add enough vodka to barely cover the herbs. Stir well, close lid securely, and allow it to stand for one week. Strain this tincture and mix it into the elderberry syrup for an elixir.

NOTE: Deanna says: "Take 1–2 tablespoons daily during cold and flu season to strengthen the immune system. During an acute cold, 1–2 tablespoons can be taken three times daily."

WHAT YOU'LL USE IT FOR:

* Immune function (for preventing colds, flu)
* Inflammation (for treating colds, flu)
* Bladder health
* Metabolic syndrome
* Cancer protection
* Prostate health
* Heart health

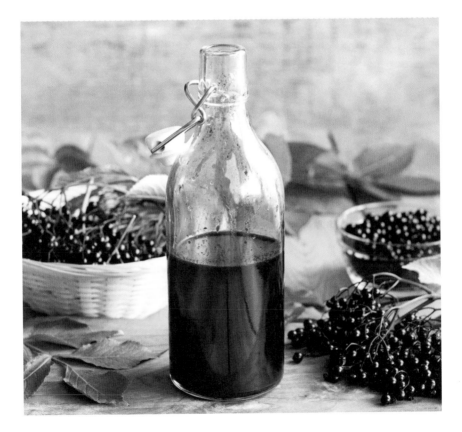

NERVE TONIC TINCTURE
Compliments of Deanna Gabriel Vierck

Deanna says: "Both skullcap and chamomile are highly valued herbs for soothing the nervous system. Skullcap has been shown to assist the body in repairing damaged tissue, and chamomile is known for being a powerful anti-inflammatory herb. If using this tincture as a digestive aide, I recommend taking it with a cup of ginger and licorice tea before or after a meal."

48 (½-teaspoon) servings

WHAT YOU'LL NEED:

¼ cup dried skullcap

¼ cup dried chamomile

1 cup 80-proof vodka

1 dose CBD alcohol- or oil-based tincture or nano-liposomal oil per 1 dose Nerve Tonic Tincture

WHAT YOU'LL DO:

1. Pour the dried skullcap and chamomile into a glass pint jar.

2. Cover the herbs completely with the vodka.

3. Shake thoroughly and leave it at room temperature for 2–4 weeks, shaking it each day.

4. Strain out the herb and pour the tincture into a dark glass bottle. The dark glass bottle allows for better storage.

5. Label the bottle with the date, the name of the tincture, and the ingredients.

6. Take 2 droppers, or ½ teaspoon, 2–3 times daily. Mix a dose of CBD supplement into each serving.

WHAT YOU'LL USE IT FOR:

* Pain (chronic and acute)

* Addiction (through anxiety and stress management)

* Asthma (through anxiety management)

* Depression (and related irritability)

* Insomnia

* Digestion (through pre-meal relaxation)

* Epilepsy and seizures (if you drop the chamomile and double the skullcap)

* Fibromyalgia

* Lyme disease

* Palliative care

* PTS

* Stress and anxiety

* Women's health

* Wound healing (from within)

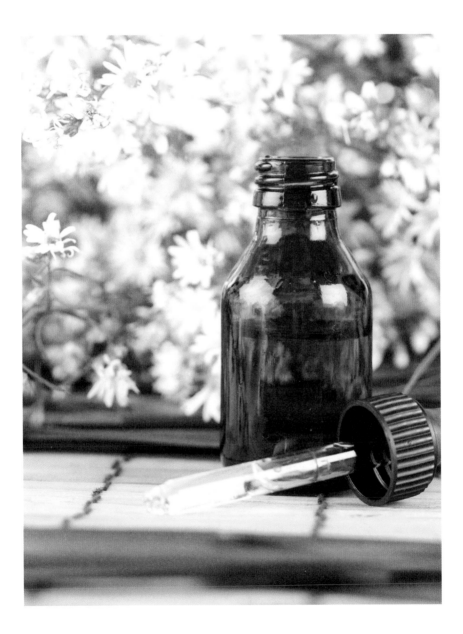

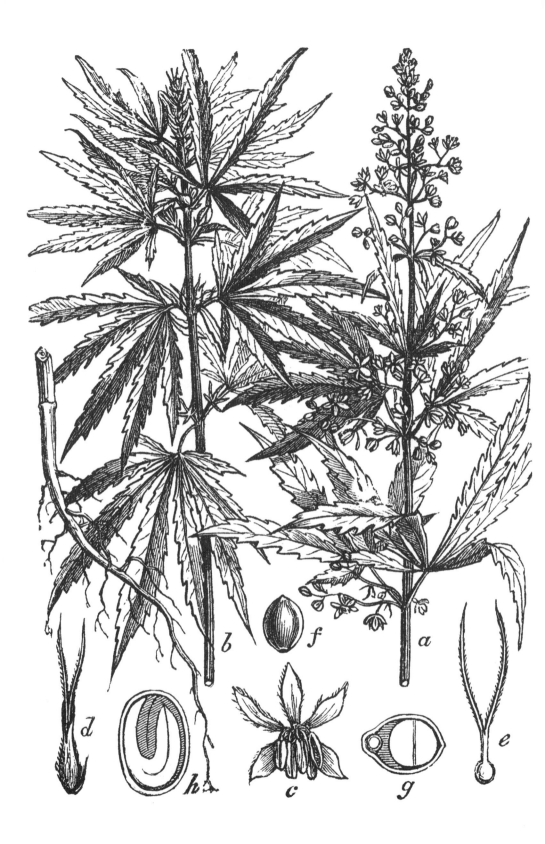

APPENDIX

GLOSSARY

AERIAL PLANT PARTS The part of the plant above ground, including the stem, leaves, flowers, and branches.

ANALGESIC Pain relieving.

ANANDAMIDE An endocannabinoid called anandamide has been found to help ease pain and depression. It may also play a role in fertility and women's health, by enhancing uterine lining and helping a fertilized egg implant and grow.

ANTI-INFLAMMATORY Acts against chemicals that cause inflamed tissue, whether in arthritic joints or from insect stings or poison ivy.

ANTIOXIDANT Prevents harmful molecules from oxidizing, or breaking down, cells and contributing to cancer, arthritis, and other diseases.

BIDIRECTIONAL EFFECT A theory that cannabinoids may adapt differently to different body endocannabinoid systems and chemistries to effect the needed change.

BIPHASIC Having two phases. Marijuana and other addictive substances, like alcohol, are biphasic; a little may be good for the body, but the "good" feeling and effect can lead to greater consumption, which is harmful.

BROAD SPECTRUM These hemp CBD products include all the phyto-cannabinoids and nutrients from the hemp plant, without any traces of THC.

CANNABINOIDS A family of healing chemical compounds produced naturally in the body as well as in hemp and marijuana plants. They interact with the endocannabinoid system to help the body maintain homeostasis. In the body, they're called endocannabinoids; in plants, they're called phytocannabinoids. Some marijuana phytocannabinoids produce a "high."

CANNABIDIOL Also called CBD. A phytocannabinoid that populates the hemp and marijuana plants and has healing effects without the "high" that is triggered by other phytocannabinoids such as THC (*see* THC). Research shows it is the most abundant of the phytocannabinoids.

CANNABIS The plant umbrella that includes CBD-rich hemp and THC-rich marijuana.

CAROTENOIDS Phytonutrients in fruits and vegetables that are antioxidant and responsible for vivid yellows and oranges in pumpkin, carrots, and other fruits and vegetables.

CBD *See* Cannabidiol

COA Certificate of Analysis. Document that gives a CBD product's origin, chemical content, and purity. Potential CBD buyers should always check a product's COA.

CONCENTRATE A pure CBD product right after it's been extracted (*see* Extraction Methods) and before it is made into a tincture or other product.

ECS *See* Endocannabinoid System

ELLAGIC ACID A phytonutrient found in strawberries and raspberries that may help protect cells against oxidation.

ENDOCANNABINOID A cannabinoid, a healing chemical compound, that is naturally produced by the body. In plants, a similar compound is called phytocannabinoid.

ENDOCANNABINOID SYSTEM Also called ECS. A bodily system that helps maintain homeostasis, or balance, in body operations such as inflammation control, and healthy brain, nerve, circulation, and immune function, among other benefits.

ENDOCANNABINOID TONE The health of the endocannabinoid system. Optimal endocannabinoid tone means that all systems are humming along, working together harmoniously, and supporting a balanced, healthy body.

ENTOURAGE EFFECT Using products made with all the plant constituents has a more powerful healing effect than using products that isolate the CBD. The more than 100 other cannabinoids in hemp support one another to increase their individual power. This yields a richer, more lasting healing effect.

EXTRACTION METHODS The processes used to remove CBD from the hemp plant CO_2, which uses carbon dioxide to pull out the CBD; ethanol, which uses alcohol; and oil. CO_2 and ethanol are considered the safest and are the most used.

FLAVONOIDS A diverse group of phytonutrients (plant nutrients) found in almost all fruits and vegetables. Along with carotenoids, they are responsible for the vivid colors in fruits and vegetables—in this case red, blue, and purple. Like carotenoids, they are antioxidant and packed with healing powers.

FREE RADICALS Unstable atoms with unpaired electrons the body generates when exposed to pollutants and disease. To stabilize, free radicals steal electrons from other molecules, causing a chain reaction of electron raiding that promotes oxidative stress, or cell damage.

FULL SPECTRUM A hemp CBD product that contains many phyto-cannabinoids and other nutrients, including the minimal THC amount (0.3 percent or less), per hemp's legal definition.

GMO Genetically modified organisms that include plants, such as corn and soy, whose natural makeup has been altered to resist insects and disease and that may contain toxins.

HEMP Also called industrial hemp, the plant under the cannabis plant umbrella that has been grown for centuries to make rope and canvas. It also carries healthful phytocannabinoids, mainly CBD.

HEMP CBD PRODUCT A product made from the hemp plant that contains more healing CBD than THC. Legal hemp CBD products contain less than 0.3 percent THC. Such products can be purchased as alcohol- or oil-based tinctures, oils, isolate powders, foods, and topical salves and balms.

HOMEOSTASIS The balance of all bodily systems for optimal function and health.

HORMONAL Supports hormone balance and endocrine system function.

ISO Be sure the manufacturer or the lab are accredited and operate according to the ISO, or International Organization for Standardization.

ISOLATE A CBD extract is refined down to a powder of pure CBD, "isolating" it from any oils, fatty acids, or other plant components that may contribute to a full-healing entourage effect. It can more quickly address certain conditions; it dissolves easily and can be used to make many products.

NANO-LIPOSOMAL OIL For a product with optimal uptake, CBD is extracted through CO_2 or ethanol (alcohol) methods; then an additional process called nano- (small) liposomal (fat-injected) makes the CBD molecules extremely small and then encloses them in a lipid, or fat, layer.

OMEGA-3 FATTY ACIDS Essential fats (ingested through diet) that support healthy heart, brain, and metabolism function.

OMEGA-6 FATTY ACIDS Essential fats (ingested through diet) that deliver energy to the body and aid in healthy inflammatory response to injury and disease. Too much, through the Western diet of polyunsaturated fats and fast foods, can trigger unhealthy inflammation that leads to disease.

OXIDATION/OXIDATIVE STRESS Cell damage caused by free radicals. It's the same process that rusts a car or turns an apple brown.

PHYTOCANNABINOIDS Some 100 kinds of healing chemical compounds (among other plant nutrients) likely produced exclusively in the hemp and marijuana plants. To date, cannabidiol, or CBD, is known to be the most abundant kind of phytocannabinoid.

PHYTONUTRIENTS Plant chemicals, or nutrients, that protect the plant from germs, fungus, and other threats, and that transfer to us through plant foods, boosting efficient body function. Examples: cannabinoids, carotenoids, ellagic acid, flavonoids, and terpenes.

RESIN Sticky, dew-like drops covering the marijuana plant, from which healing components are extracted to make medicine; hemp is not as rich in resin as is marijuana.

SUBLINGUAL DELIVERY Meaning delivery "under the tongue," this method is recommended for optimal uptake when administering CBD products through droppers or pumps.

TERPENES Including limonene and pinene, they are responsible for the aroma of cannabis and for fighting unhealthy inflammation and cell deterioration. They also are natural bug repellents, especially limonene.

TETRAHYDROCANNABINOL Also called THC. A phytocannabinoid in the hemp and marijuana plants that both heals and, in large concentration, causes a "high," or psychoactivity.

THC (*SEE* TETRAHYDROCANNABINOL)

TITRATION Starting at a low medicine dosage and gradually building up to determine its optimal healing effect on the body.

TINCTURE Delivery system for CBD. Plant parts are soaked in ethanol (alcohol) to extract the active healing ingredients. Final products are either as a straight alcohol tincture or diluted with oil (oil-based alcohol tincture) or glycerine (glycerine-based alcohol tincture) for less potent delivery.

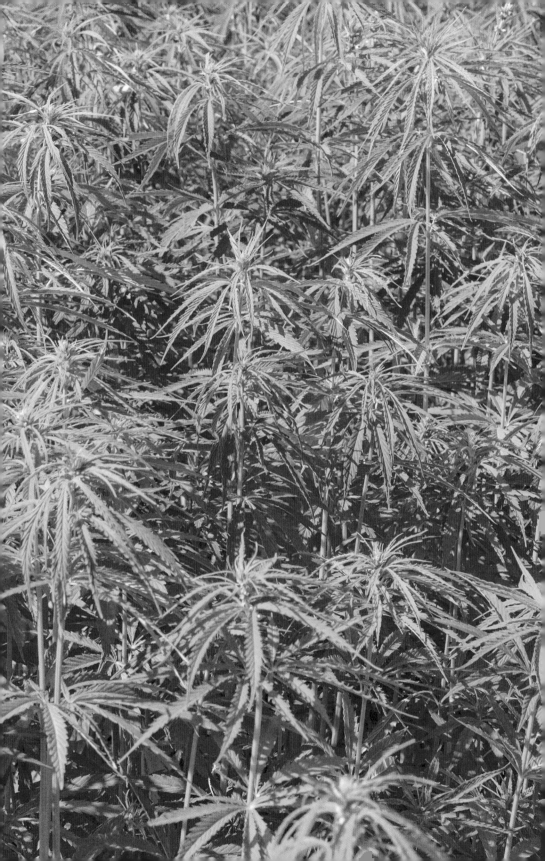

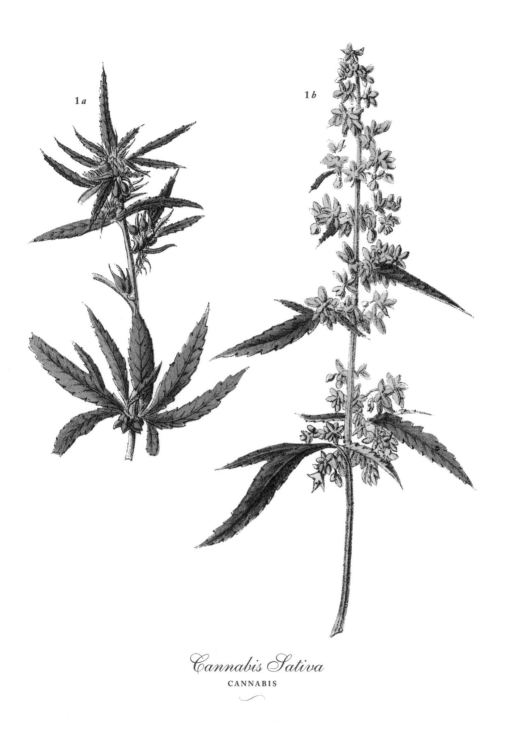

1 *a*

1 *b*

Cannabis Sativa

CANNABIS

FURTHER READING

BOOKS

Backes, Michael, with J. McCue, M.D., ed. *Cannabis Pharmacy: The Practical Guide to Medical Marijuana*, New York: Black Dog & Leventhal Publishers, 2014.

Booth, Martin. *Cannabis: A History*. New York: Picador, 2005.

Brownell Grogan, Barbara. *Healing Herbs Handbook: Recipes for Natural Living*. New York: Sterling, 2018.

Dean, Carolyn, M.D., N.D., et al., eds. *1,801 Home Remedies: Trustworthy Treatments for Everyday Health Problems*. New York: Reader's Digest, 2004.

Holland, Julie, ed. *The Pot Book: A Complete Guide to Cannabis, Its Role in Medicine, Politics, Science, and Culture*. Rochester, VT: Park Street Press, 2010.

Gladstar, Rosemary. *Rosemary Gladstar's Herbal Recipes for Vibrant Health: 175 Teas, Tonics, Oils, Salves, Tinctures, and Other Natural Remedies for the Entire Family*. North Adams, MA: Storey Publishing, 2008.

Graedon, Joe, and T. Graedon. *National Geographic Complete Guide to Natural Home Remedies: 1,025 Easy Ways to Live Longer, Feel Better, and Enrich Your Life*. Washington, DC: National Geographic, 2011.

Lee, Martin. *Smoke Signals: A Social History of Marijuana—Medical, Recreational, and Scientific*. New York, NY: Scribner, 2012.

Leinow, Leonard, J. Birnbaum, and Michael H. Moskowitz, M.D., foreword. *CBD: A Patient's Guide to Medicinal Cannabis, Healing Without the High*. Berkeley, CA: North Atlantic Books, 2017.

Lidicker, Gretchen. *CBD Oil Everyday Secrets: A Lifestyle Guide to Hemp-Derived Health and Wellness*. New York: The Countryman Press, W.W. Norton, 2018.

Low Dog, Tieroana, M.D., D. Kiefer, M.D., R. Johnson, and S. Foster. *National Geographic Guide to Medicinal Herbs: The World's Most Effective Healing Plants*. Washington, DC: National Geographic, 2011.

Mindell, Earl, RPH, MH, PhD. *Healing with Hemp CBD Oil: A Simple Guide to Using Powerful and Proven Health Benefits of CBD*. Garden City Park, NY: Square One Publishers, 2018.

Rappaport, Tina, BFA, and S. Leonard-Johnson, RN, PhD. *CBD-Rich Hemp Oil: Cannabis Medicine Is Back.* Scotts Valley, CA: CreateSpace, 2014.

Russo, Ethan. "The Pharmacological History of Cannabis." In *Handbook of Cannabinoids,* R. Pertwee, ed. Oxford, UK: Oxford University Press, 2014.

Shealy, Norman. *The Illustrated Encyclopedia of Healing Remedies.* New York: Harper Element, 2002.

White, Linda B., Barbara H. Seeber, and Barbara Brownell Grogan. *500 Time-Tested Home Remedies and the Science Behind Them.* Beverly, MA: Fair Winds Press, 2013.

White, Linda B., and Steven Foster. *The Herbal Drugstore: The Best Natural Alternatives to Over-the-Counter and Prescription Medicines.* Emmaus, PA: Rodale, 2003.

Yeager, Selene, and the editors of *Prevention. The Doctors Book of Food Remedies.* Emmaus, PA: Rodale, 2007.

WEBSITES

Charlotte's Web: Stanley Brothers: https://www.cwhemp.com

Healthline: https://www.healthline.com

Leafly: Cannabis 101, Growing, Strains, Politics, Health, Lifestyle, Science and Tech: https://www.leafly.com

Marijuana Business Daily: https://mjbizdaily.com

Mayo Clinic: https://www.mayoclinic.org

Medicine Hunter: http://www.medicinehunter.com

Mind Body Green: https://www.mindbodygreen.com

Ministry of Hemp: https://ministryofhemp.com

National Conference of State Legislatures on State Industrial Hemp Statutes: http://www.ncsl.org/research/agriculture-and-rural-development/state-industrial-hemp-statutes.aspx

National Hemp Association: https://nationalhempassociation.org

National Institutes of Health Library of Medicine: https://www.nlm.nih.gov

National Institute on Drug Abuse: Advancing Addiction Science: https://www.drugabuse.gov

Naturally Recovering Autism, https://naturallyrecoveringautism.com

Project CBD: Medical Marijuana and Cannabinoid Science: https://www.projectcbd.org

U.S. Food and Drug Administration: https://www.fda.gov

Web MD: https://www.webmd.com

VIDEOS

Lee, Martin. "Interview with Dr. Ethan Russo: CBD, the Entourage Effect, and the Microbiome." Project CBD, 2019, at https://www.projectcbd.org/dr-ethan-russo-cbd-entourage-effect-and-microbiome.

Lee, Martin. "From Clone to Concentrate: How CBD Oil Is Made." Project CBD, 2017, at https://www.projectcbd.org/about/herbal-medicine/clone-concentrate-how-cbd-oil-made.

Thomas, Karen. "Interview with Dr. Christopher Shade: How to Get the Greatest Nutritional Absorption with Lowered Dosages." Naturally Recovering Autism, 2018, at https://naturallyrecoveringautism.com/2018/02/28/get-greatest-nutritional-absorption-lowered-dosages/.

SELECTED ARTICLES

Al, Idris. "Cannabinoid Receptors as Target for Treatment of Osteoporosis." *Current Neuropharmacology*, 2010, at https://www.ncbi.nlm.nih.gov/pubmed/21358974.

Andre, C., et. al, "Cannabis Sativa: The Plant of One Thousand Molecules." *Frontiers in Plant Science*, 2016, at https://www.ncbi.nlm.nih.gov/pmc/articles/PMC4740396.

Appendino, G., et al. "Antibacterial Cannabinoids from Cannabis Sativa." *Journal of Natural Products*, at https://www.ncbi.nlm.nih.gov/pubmed/18681481.

Bar-Sela, G., et al. "The Medical Necessity for Medicinal Cannabis: … Treatment in Cancer Patients on Supportive or Palliative Care." *Evidence-Based Complementary Alternative Medicine*, 2017, at https://www.ncbi.nlm.nih.gov/pubmed/23956774.

Bitencourt, R., and R. Takahashi "Cannabidiol as a Therapeutic Alternative for Post-Traumatic Stress Disorder." *Frontiers in Neuroscience*, 2018, at https://www.ncbi.nlm.nih.gov/pmc/articles/PMC6066583/.

Booz, G. W. "Cannabidiol as an Emergent Therapeutic Strategy for Lessening the Impact of Oxidative Stress." *Free Radical Biology & Medicine*, 2011, at https://www.ncbi.nlm.nih.gov/pubmed/21238581.

Bridgeman, M., et al. "Medicinal Cannabis: History, Pharmacology, and Implications for the Acute Care Setting" *Pharmacy and Therapeutics*, 2017, at https://www.ncbi.nlm.nih.gov/pmc/articles/PMC5312634/.

Campbell, C. " Cannabinoids in Pediatrics" *Journal of Pediatric Pharmacology and Therapeutics*, 2017, at https://www.ncbi.nlm.nih.gov/pmc/articles/PMC5473390/.

Corroon, J., and J. A. Phillips "A Cross-Sectional Study of Cannabidiol Users" *Cannabis and Cannabinoid Research*, 2018, at https://www.ncbi.nlm.nih.gov/pubmed/30014038.

Darkovska-Serafimoskva, M., et al. "Pharmacotherapeutic Considerations for Use of Cannabinoids to Relieve Pain in Patients with Malignant Diseases." *Journal of Pain Research*, at https://www.ncbi.nlm.nih.gov/pmc/articles/PMC5922297/.

Dmietrieva, N. "Endocannabinoid Involvement in Endometriosis." *Pain*, 2010, at https://www.ncbi.nlm.nih.gov/pubmed/20833475.

Grill, M., et al., "Medical Cannabis and Cannabinoids: An Option for the Treatment of Inflammatory Bowel Disease and Cancer of the Colon?" *Medical Cannabis and Cannabinoids*, 2018, at https://www.karger.com/Article/FullText/489036.

Grill, M. et al. "Cellular Localization and Regulation of Receptors and Enzymes of the Endocannabinoid System in Intestinal and Systemic Inflammation." *Histochemistry and Cell Biology*, 2019, at https://www.ncbi.nlm.nih.gov/pubmed/30196316.

Gumbiner, J., PhD. "History of Cannabis in India." *Psychology Today*, 2011, at https://www.psychologytoday.com/us/blog/the-teenage-mind/201106/history-cannabis-in-india.

Habib, G., and S. Artul. "Medical Cannabis for the Treatment of Fibromyalgia." *Journal of Clinical Rheumatology*, 2018, at https://www.ncbi.nlm.nih.gov/pubmed/29461346.

Hammell, D. C., et al. "Transdermal Cannabidiol Reduces Inflammation and Pain-Related Behaviors in a Rat Model of Arthritis." *European Journal of Pain*, 2015, at https://www.ncbi.nlm.nih.gov/pubmed/26517407.

Hilliard, C. J., and Q. S. Liu. "Endocannabinoid Signaling in the Etiology and Treatment of Depressive Illness." *Current Pharmaceutical Design*, 2014, at https://www.ncbi.nlm.nih.gov/pubmed/24180398.

Horvath, B., et al. "The Endocannabinoid System and Plant-Derived Cannabinoids in Diabetes and Diabetic Complications." *The American Journal of Pathology*, 2012, at https://www.ncbi.nlm.nih.gov/pmc/articles/PMC3349875/.

Huang, W. "Endocannabinoid System: Role in Depression, Reward, and Pain Control." *Molecular Medicine Reports*, 2016, at https://www.ncbi.nlm.nih.gov/pmc/articles/PMC5042796/.

Iffland, K. "An Update on Safety and Side Effects of Cannabidiol: A Review of Clinical Data and Relevant Animal Studies." *Cannabis and Cannabinoid Research*, 2017, at https://www.ncbi.nlm.nih.gov/pmc/articles/PMC5569602/.

Johnson, J. "Everything You Need to Know About CBD Oil." *Medical News Today*, 2018, at https://www.medicalnewstoday.com/articles/317221.php.

Kelly, C., et al. "Distinct Effects of Childhood ADHD and Cannabis Use on Brain Functional Architecture in Young Adults." *Neuroimage: Clinical*, 2017, at https://www.ncbi.nlm.nih.gov/pmc/articles/PMC5153452/.

Kinderlehrer, D. "Can Medical Marijuana Help Treat Lyme Disease? A Doctor's Perspective." LymeDisease.org News, at https://www.lymedisease.org/med-marijuana-lyme-kinderlehrer/.

Kogan, N. "Cannabinoids in Health and Disease." *Dialogues in Clinical Neuroscience*, 2007, at https://www.ncbi.nlm.nih.gov/pmc/articles/PMC3202504/.

Lee, M. "No Brainer: CBD and THC for Head Injuries." *Project CBD*, 2018, at https://www.projectcbd.org/science/no-brainer-cbd-and-thc-head-injuries.

Linge, R. "Cannabidiol Induces Rapid-Acting Antidepressant-like Effects...." *Neuropharmacology*, 2016, at https://www.ncbi.nlm.nih.gov/pubmed/26711860.

Lochte, B., et al. "The Use of Cannabis for Headache Disorders." *Cannabis and Cannabinoid Research*, 2017, at https://www.ncbi.nlm.nih.gov/pmc/articles/PMC5436334/.

Lowe, H., et al. "Potential of Cannabidiol for the Treatment of Viral Hepatitis." *Pharmacognosy Research*, 2017, at https://www.ncbi.nlm.nih.gov/pmc/articles/PMC5330095/.

Marco, E., et al. "The Role of the Endocannabinoid System in Eating Disorders." *Behavioral Pharmacology*, 2012, at https://www.ncbi.nlm.nih.gov/pubmed/22785439.

Marcu, J. "CBD and Epilepsy." Project CBD, 2014, at https://www.projectcbd.org/about/clinical-research/cbd-and-epilepsy.

McAllister, S., et al. "The Anti-Tumor Activity of Plant-Derived Non-Psychoactive Cannabinoids." *Journal of Neuroimmune Pharmacology*, 2015, at https://www.ncbi.nlm.nih.gov/pmc/articles/PMC4470774/.

McGuire, P. "Cannabidiol (CBD) as an Adjunctive Therapy in Schizophrenia: A Multicenter Randomized Controlled Trial" *American Journal of Psychiatry*, 2018, at https://www.ncbi.nlm.nih.gov/pubmed/29241357.

Morena, M. et al., "Neurobiological Interactions Between Stress and the Endocannabinoid System," *Neuropsychopharmacology*, 2016, at https://www.ncbi.nlm.nih.gov/pubmed/26068727.

Murillo-Rodriguez, E., et al. "Potential Effects of Cannabidiol as a Wake-Promoting Agent" *Current Neuropharmacology*, 2014, at https://www.ncbi.nlm.nih.gov/pmc/articles/PMC4023456/.

Nagarkatti, P., et al. "Cannabinoids as Novel Anti-Inflammatory Drugs." *Future Medicinal Chemistry*, 2009, at https://www.ncbi.nlm.nih.gov/pmc/articles/PMC2828614/.

National Hemp Association "Cannabinoids as Antioxidants and Neuroprotectants" (abstract for Hemp U.S. Patent Number 6,630,507, 2016), at https://nationalhempassociation.org/cannabinoids-as-antioxidants-and-neuroprotectants/.

Olah, A., et al. "Cannabidiol Exerts Sebostatic and Anti-inflammatory Effects on Human Sebocytes.", *Journal of Clinical Investigation*, 2014, at https://www.ncbi.nlm.nih.gov/pubmed/25061872.

Parker, L. "Regulation of Nausea and Vomiting by Cannabinoids." *British Journal of Pharmacology*, 2011, at https://www.ncbi.nlm.nih.gov/pmc/articles/PMC3165951/.

Pava, M. J., et al. "Endocannabinoid Signaling Regulates Sleep Stability." *PLOS-One*, 2016, at https://www.ncbi.nlm.nih.gov/pmc/articles/PMC4816426/.

Peres, F. F., et al., "Cannabidiol as a Promising Strategy to Treat and Prevent Movement Disorders?" *Frontiers of Pharmacology*, 2018, at https://www.ncbi.nlm.nih.gov/pubmed/29867488.

Pertwee, R. G. "Cannabinoid Pharmacology: The First 66 Years." *British Journal of Pharmacology*, 2006, at https://www.ncbi.nlm.nih.gov/pubmed/16402100.

Pini, A. "The Role of Cannabinoids in Inflammatory Modulation of Allergic Respiratory Disorders, Inflammatory Pain, and Ischemic Stroke." *Current Drug Targets*, 2012, at https://www.ncbi.nlm.nih.gov/pubmed/22420307.

Piomelli, D., and E. B. Russo. "The *Cannabis sativa* Versus *Cannabis indica* Debate: An Interview with Ethan Russo, MD." *Cannabis and Cannabinoid Research*, 2016, at https://www.ncbi.nlm.nih.gov/pmc/articles/PMC5576603/.

Reiss, C. "Cannabinoids and Viral Infections." *Pharmaceuticals*, 2010, at https://www.ncbi.nlm.nih.gov/pmc/articles/PMC2903762/.

Rudroff, T. "Cannabidiol to Improve Mobility in People with Multiple Sclerosis." *Frontiers in Neurology*, 2018, at https://www.ncbi.nlm.nih.gov/pmc/articles/PMC5874292/.

Russo, Ethan. "Clinical Endocannabinoid Deficiency Reconsidered: Current Research Supports Theory in Migraine, Fibromyalgia, Irritable Bowel, and Other Treatment-Resistant Syndromes." *Cannabis Cannabinoid Research*, 2016, at https://www.ncbi.nlm.nih.gov/pubmed/28861491.

Russo, Ethan. "Introduction to the Endocannabinoid System." Phytecs, 2015, at https://www.phytecs.com/wp-content/uploads/2015/02/IntroductionECS.pdf.

Russo, Ethan. "Taming THC: Potential Cannabis Synergy and Phytocannabinoid-Terpenoid Entourage Effects." *British Journal of Pharmacology*, 2011, at https://www.ncbi.nlm.nih.gov/pmc/articles/PMC3165946/.

Russo, Ethan, and Andrea G. Hohmann. "Role of Cannabinoids in Pain Management." In *Comprehensive Treatment of Chronic Pain by Medical, Interventional, and Behavioral Approaches*. New York: Springer, 2013.

Sharma, M., et al. "In Vitro Anticancer Activity of Plant-Derived Cannabidiol on Prostate Cancer Cell Lines." *Pharmacology and Pharmacy*, 2014, at https://file.scirp.org/Html/5-2500510_47691.htm.

Stanley C. "Is the Cardiovascular System a Therapeutic Target for Cannabidiol?" *British Journal of Clinical Pharmacology*, 2013, at https://www.ncbi.nlm.nih.gov/pmc/articles/PMC3579247/.

Thapa, D. "The Cannabinoids Δ8THC, CBD, and HU-308 Act via Distinct Receptors to Reduce Corneal Pain and Inflammation." *Cannabis and Cannabinoid Research*, 2018, at https://www.ncbi.nlm.nih.gov/pmc/articles/PMC5812319/.

Tibirica, E. "The Multiple Functions of the Endocannabinoid System: A Focus on the Regulation of Food Intake." *Diabetology and Metabolic Syndrome*, at https://www.ncbi.nlm.nih.gov/pmc/articles/PMC2832623/.

Turcotte, C. "Impact of Cannabis, Cannabinoids, and Endocannabinoids in the Lungs." *Frontiers of Pharmacology*, 2016, at https://www.ncbi.nlm.nih.gov/pmc/articles/PMC5023687/.

U.S. Food and Drug Administration. "FDA Approves First Drug Comprised of an Active Ingredient Derived from Marijuana to Treat Rare, Severe Forms of Epilepsy." FDA News Release, June 25, 2018, at https://www.fda.gov/newsevents/newsroom/pressannouncements/ucm611046.htm.

Wang, Z., et al. "Treatment with a Cannabinoid Receptor 2 Agonist Decreases Severity of Established Cystitis." *Journal of Urology*, 2013, at https://www.jurology.com/article/S0022-5347(13)05841-2/abstract.

Yang, Y., et al. "*Cannabis Sativa* (Hemp) Seeds, Tetrahydrocannabinal, and Potential Overdose." *Cannabis and Cannabinoid Research*, 2017, at https://www.ncbi.nlm.nih.gov/pmc/articles/PMC5665515/.

Yin, J., et al. "Biocompatible Nanoemulsions Based on Hemp Oil and Less Surfactants for Oral Delivery of Baicalein with Enhanced Bioavailablility." *International Journal of Nanomedicine*, 2017, at https://www.ncbi.nlm.nih.gov/pmc/articles/PMC5391827/.

Young, S. "Marijuana Stops Child's Severe Seizures." CNN Report, August 7, 2013, at https://www.cnn.com/2013/08/07/health/charlotte-child-medical-marijuana/index.html.

ACKNOWLEDGMENTS

Sharing the story and power of CBD has been a pleasure and a privilege. I'd like to thank Sterling editor Nicole Fisher for bringing this "hot topic" to me, and for her vision and guidance in presenting it with simplicity and clarity. My hope is that the book and its research will spark further questions and the desire to learn more about cannabis—an extraordinary natural healer. Thank you to the Sterling team—Elysia Liang, Ellina Litmanovich, Linda Liang, Christine Heun, and Elizabeth Lindy.

Consultant Deanna Gabriel Vierck brought to the project her expertise as a clinical herbalist, nutritionist, and flower essence practitioner—and her heart and soul. I am grateful for her knowledge, scientific yet friendly approach, and can-do attitude; and for our weekly sessions packed with her solid information, wisdom, and laughter. Each page bears Deanna's influence and that of my integrative nutrition mentor Dr. Linda B. White, with whom I wrote a book and many articles on natural remedies before she passed away in 2015.

Jahnna Beecham, friend, editorial colleague, and coauthor of *Living with Dying*, lent her knowledge, support, and contacts; Barclay Walsh, NPR researcher and friend, introduced me to Chris Walsh, founding editor and president of *Marijuana Business Daily*, who gave key guidance on the future of the cannabis industry; Laura Soto-Barra, NPR chief archivist and friend, shared many insightful books on the power of plants; Tammy Sweet, codirector of Heartstone Center for Earth Essentials underscored the importance of the cannabis plant and the need to share information about it; Rosemary Gladstar, founder of Sage Mountain Retreat Center and Native Plant Preserve sponsored the first Medicinal Cannabis Conference on the East Coast, in which luminaries including Dr. Ethan Russo, neurologist and director of research and development for the International Cannabis and Cannabinoids Institute; Dr. Dustin Sulak, integrative medicine practitioner and founder of Healer.com; and Chris Kilham, founder of Medicine Hunter, Inc. shared their research and practical experiences reflected in this book.

Thank you to Katja Swift and Ryn Midura of the Commonwealth Center for Holistic Herbalism for their insight on Lyme disease, and to Lynn Brownell and Katie Brownell, Julia Kay, Amy Ellis of Color Cuisine, and Ashley Sarkozy of Botanical Roots, for sharing their recipes. Thanks to all who gave testimonials about their experiences using CBD: Ben Cardamone, Katie Ortlip (coauthor of *Living with Dying*), Sarah McNaughton, Skye Hillgartner, and Maggie McLaughlin. I am grateful to my extended family and friends, who cheered me on and participated in evening tasting/critique sessions, and to my immediate family— Dan, Meredith, William, and Caroline—who support me always, in every way.

INDEX

IMAGE CREDITS

ALAMY: Pixel-shot: 165

DEPOSITPHOTOS.COM: ©5PHL
150; ©imagepointfr: 183; ©Kostrez: 28;
©liudmilachernetska@gmail.com: 197;
©Natalya.stepowaya: 162; ©neillangan:
159; ©Pinkyone: 156; ©Tinnakorn: vi

GETTY IMAGES: DigitalVision
Vectors: bauhause1000: 212;
ilbusca: 206; iStock/Getty Images
Plus: Artfully79: 198; baibaz: 146;
Roman Bykhalets: 15 right; Marcus
Calvo: 22; danathefox: 193; Erpeewee:
211; FabrikaCr: 38; Foxys_forest_
manufacutre: 132; instamatics: 152;
jessicahyde: 25; juankphoto: 205;
Julia_Sudnitskaya: 167; Kenshi991: 15
left ; laartist: 138; Madeleine_Steinbach:
203; MysteryShot: 135; nadisja: 201;
NataGolubnycha: 49; NoSystem Images:
55; pidjoe: 168; rezkrr: ii; RyanKing999:
84; tashka2000: 155; tiverylucky: 142;
tomazi: 68

LIBRARY OF CONGRESS: 12, 27

SHUTTERSTOCK.COM: elenabsl: 7;
Eskymaks: 60; photopixel: 113

STOCKFOOD: ©Boguslaw Bialy;
©Brigitte Sporrer: 179

STOCKSY UNITED: ©Canan
Czemmel: 141; ©Davide Illini: 97;
©Studio Firma: 191

WELLCOME COLLECTION: x, 9, 10

**COURTESY OF WIKIMEDIA
COMMONS:** 4

ABOUT THE AUTHOR

BARBARA BROWNELL GROGAN is former editor-in-chief of National Geographic Books and a certified health coach through New York's Institute for Integrative Nutrition. At National Geographic, she grew the health and body line of reference books with titles including *Nature's Medicine, Brainworks, Body: The Complete Human, Medicinal Herbs,* and *The People's Pharmacy: Quick and Handy Home Remedies.* She is coauthor of *500 Time-Tested Home Remedies and the Science Behind Them* (Fair Winds Press, 2013) and *Healing Herbs Handbook* (Sterling, 2018), and editor for the USDA'S *Guide to Infant Nutrition* (USDA, 2018). From 2013 to 2018, she coauthored the integrative nutrition column Remedy Chicks at Everyday Health.